CW00469406

THE KETO DIET

FOR

BEGINNERS:

GAIN COMPLETE CLARITY ON KETOGENIC
DIET LIFESTYLE

PAULA NASH

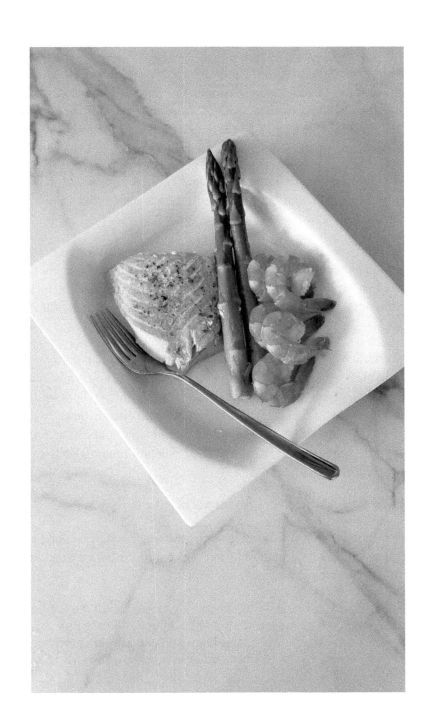

TABLE OF CONTENTS

THE KETO DIET FOR BEGINNERS: i

Introduction 1

Chapter 1: Introduction to the ketogenic diet 3

WHAT IS THE KETOGENIC DIET? 3

HOW KETOGENIC DIET IS DIFFERENT FROM OTHER LOW-CARB DIETS 7

KETO DIET'S HISTORY 8

WHAT IS KETOSIS? 9

ADAPTATION STEPS OF OUR BODY TO KETOSIS 9

TYPES OF KETOSIS 11

Carbohydrate-Restricted Ketosis 11

Supplemental Ketosis 12

Fasting Ketosis 12

SIGNS YOU ARE IN KETOSIS 12

Dry Mouth 13

Increased Urination 13

Ketone Scent 13

Loss of Hunger 13

HOW TO MEASURE KETONES 14

Judging from Symptoms of Ketosis 14

Urine Strips 14

Breath Analyzer. 15

Blood Ketone Meter. 16

HOW TO ENTER KETOSIS 16

Chapter 2: How Metabolism Works when you are on the ketogenic diet
.... 19

METABOLIC EFFECTS OF THE KETOGENIC DIET 20

MACRONUTRIENTS BREAK DOWN 21

Carb Intake 22

Protein Intake 22

Fat Intake 22

FATS AND CARBS IN THE KETO DIET 23

CARBOHYDRATE LOADING 24

HOW TO BALANCE YOUR HORMONES ON A KETO DIET? 27

Chapter 3: Ketogenic Diet and Weight Loss 31

How does Ketogenic diet help you lose weight? 33
Some Common Weight Loss Principles to Note 34
    Weigh Your Food 34
    Keep hunger at bay 35
    Be sustainable 36
    Exercise 36
    Reduce Your Stress 37
    Choose Quality Carbs 37
    Stay Away from Diet Soda 37
    Get Enough Sleep 37
    Intermittent Fasting: 38
Sports and Keto Diet? 38

Chapter 4: Clarifying the common Myths about the Ketogenic Diet.....41
Carbohydrates as an essential macronutrient 41
Ketogenic diet is dangerous because of Ketosis 41
There will be tremendous damage for your kidneys because of
    high Protein consumption 42
The ketogenic diet is just a fad diet 42
The ketogenic diet is hard to stick to 43
The ketogenic diet will ruin your physical performance 43
Ketosis is a damaging metabolic state 44
Low Carb intake causes muscles to shrink 44
The ketogenic diet is bad for your heart 45
Most weight loss comes from water weight 45
Ketogenic Dieters suffer from low fiber intake caused disease 46

Chapter 5: What to Eat and what to avoid under Low Carb Ketogenic
diet 47
What to consume and what to avoid when switching to
    Ketogenic diets 47
    Meat 48
    Fish 48
    Eggs 48
    Natural fats and high fat sauces 48
    Vegetables cultivated above the ground 48
    Dairy foods 49
    Nuts and seeds 49
    Berries 49
    liquids 50

WHAT TO AVOID IN KETOGENIC DIETING?..50
   Sugar...*50*
   Starch..*50*
   Margarine..*51*
   Fruits...*51*

Chapter 6: Benefits of the Ketogenic Diet..................................**53**
   KETOGENIC DIET HELPS BUILD MORE LEAN MUSCLES WHILE LOSING FAT....53
   KETOGENIC DIETS INCREASE THE AMOUNT OF HDL CHOLESTEROLS WHILE
      REDUCING LDL CHOLESTEROL LEVELS...53
   CONTROL OF BLOOD SUGAR...54
   INCREASED ENERGY...54
   WEIGHT LOSS..54
   INCREASE LIFESPAN..55
   INCREASED BRAIN FUNCTION...55
   MITOCHONDRIAL FUNCTION..55
   ENERGY..56
   DIGESTIVE HEALTH BOOSTER...56
   ENDURANCE PERFORMANCE...57
   OVERALL HEALTH BENEFITS...57
   IMPROVED MENTAL FOCUS...57
   REDUCED CRAVINGS AND HUNGER PAINS...58
   CLEARER SKIN...58

Chapter 7: Adverse Effects of the Ketogenic Diet....................**61**
   HYPOGLYCEMIA..61
   Side Effects of Hypoglycemia..*62*
   Strategies for Overcoming Hypoglycemia...*63*
   HPA AXIS DYSFUNCTION..63
   Side Effects of HPA Axis Dysfunction...*64*
   Strategies for Supporting your HPA Axis...*65*
   MINERAL AND ELECTROLYTE DEFICIENCY...65
   Side Effects of Mineral and Electrolyte Deficiency Urination..................*66*
   KETOACIDOSIS...67
   Causes of Ketoacidosis...*68*
   Treatment for Ketoacidosis...*68*
   CHALLENGES IN YOUR LIFESTYLE...69
   Stress..*69*
   Sleep Deprivation...*70*
   Maintaining Your Good Work...*71*

Chapter 8: Optimizing exercise on the ketogenic diet. 73

EXERCISING FOR FAT LOSS ON THE KETOGENIC DIET 73

EXERCISING FOR MUSCLE GROWTH AND MUSCLE STRENGTH 74

TYPES OF EXERCISE ON A KETO DIET 76

    Yoga...76

    Cycling 77

    Walking 77

    Cross Fit 77

    Rowing 77

    Heavy Weight Lifting/Power Lifting 78

    Swimming 78

    High Intensity Training..78

SOME TIPS TO GET YOU MOTIVATED!...............................79

    Give your body time to adjust. 79

    Do not try any new workouts when you're starting a keto diet..............79

    Make sure you're eating enough fat. 79

    Skip high intensity workouts until you are fully adjusted to keto.............80

    Don't under eat!..80

    Don't slam your body with unnecessary calories.............81

    Spread out your workouts. 81

    Remind yourself of all the other positives of working out. 81

    Listen to your body and your doctor. 82

Chapter 9: Ketogenic diet and common diseases 83

KETO DIET AND CANCER 83

KETO DIET AND IBS (IRRITABLE BOWEL SYNDROME).............85

KETO DIET AND BLOOD SUGAR 85

KETO DIET AND ACNE 86

KETO AND EYESIGHT 87

KETO DIET AND ALZHEIMER'S 88

KETO DIET AND AUTISM...88

KETO DIET AND GERD (GASTRO ESOPHAGEAL REFLUX DISEASE).............88

KETO DIET AND HEADACHES AND MIGRAINES 88

KETO DIET AND EPILEPSY 89

KETO DIET AND BLOOD PRESSURE 89

Chapter 10: How to Make a Menu of Keto Diet? 91

GROCERY LIST FOR YOUR PERFECT KETO PLAN 91

    Fats 91

    Vegetables 91

Proteins 92

Dairy Products 93

Spices 94

Sweets 94

Sauces 95

Drinks 95

HOW TO MAKE THE MENU? 96

FEATURES OF KETO DIET FOR VEGANS 98

Chapter 11: Mistakes That Can Keep You from Being Successful on Your Ketogenic Diet 103

USING THE KETO DIET AS A "QUICK FIX" DIET METHOD 103

NOT REPLENISHING YOUR BODY'S SODIUM LEVELS 104

CONSUMING TOO MUCH PROTEIN 104

CONSUMING MORE CARBS THAN RECOMMENDED LEVELS 105

NOT BEING PATIENT 105

BEING AFRAID TO EAT FAT (EATING HIGH FAT DIETS) 106

TRYING TO IMPOSE TOO MANY CHANGES AT ONCE 106

BEING AFRAID OF EATING HIGH-FAT CONTENT 107

OBSESSING OVER YOUR WEIGHT 107

NOT TRANSITIONING SLOWLY ENOUGH TO THE DIET 107

OBSESSING ABOUT YOUR KETONE LEVELS 108

EATING THE WRONG FATS 108

FOCUSING SOLELY ON ELIMINATING CARBS 108

OVEREATING PROTEIN 109

NOT EATING SUFFICIENT AMOUNTS OF FAT 109

OVEREATING PROCESSED FOODS 110

NOT GETTING SUFFICIENT SALT, MINERALS AND VITAMINS 110

CONSUMING TOO MUCH ALCOHOL 110

EATING ON TOO RIGID OF A SCHEDULE 110

NOT COMMITTING YOURSELF FULLY TO THE DIET 111

OBSESSING ABOUT YOUR CHOLESTEROL LEVELS 111

BELIEVING THE KETO DIET IS A QUICK FIX 111

NOT BEING PREPARED FOR THE ONSET OF KETOSIS 111

COMPARING YOUR PROGRESS TO OTHERS 112

ALLOWING SETBACKS IN YOUR PROGRESS TO IMPEDE FURTHER PROGRESS 112

NOT FASTING AT ALL 113

NOT GETTING PROPER EXERCISE 113

NOT DRINKING ENOUGH WATER 113

LIVING A SEDENTARY LIFESTYLE 113
YOU'RE NOT INTRODUCING A VARIETY OF FOODS TO YOUR DIET.............114
NOT KNOWING YOUR MACROS...114
AVOIDING FIBER...114
NOT DEALING WITH STRESS..115
EATING TOO MANY NUTS 115
EATING TOO MUCH DAIRY...115
EATING PRODUCTS THAT ARE LABELED "LOW CARB" 116
DRINKING BULLETPROOF COFFEE 116
NOT PLANNING YOUR MEALS..116
NOT GETTING ENOUGH EXERCISE...116
HAVING CHEAT MEALS 117

Chapter 12: Tips to Embrace a Keto Lifestyle 119
STICK TO 30-100 GRAMS OF NET CARBS PER DAY.................................119
DETERMINE A CALORIE LEVEL THAT'S RIGHT FOR YOU. 119
CLEAN OUT THE CUPBOARDS 120
CREATE A NEW KETO GROCERY LIST 120
STOCK UP YOUR KETO KITCHEN..120
PLAN OUT YOUR FIRST WEEK'S WORTH OF MEALS 121
WHAT'S YOUR SCHEDULE? 121
FOCUS ON EATING WHAT YOU LOVE..122
TRY DIFFERENT FLAVOR COMBINATIONS 123
USE KETO STICKS OR STRIPS..123
MONITOR ANY SIDE EFFECTS YOU MIGHT EXPERIENCE DURING THE EARLY
   STAGES OF THE DIET. 124
TEST YOUR KETONE LEVELS AND COMPARE THE RESULTS TO YOUR MEAL
   CHOICES. 124
STAY HYDRATED 125
COUNT YOUR CARBS. 125
GET RID OF THOSE CARBS! 126
KEEP KETO FRIENDLY SNACKS ON HAND..126
BE PREPARED FOR WHEN YOU'RE EATING OUT. 126
START EXERCISING. 127

Chapter 13: Your 14 Day Meal Plan 129

Chapter 14: 14 Day Shopping List...133
WEEK 1..133
   Shopping list...133
WEEK 2..134

Shopping list *134*

Chapter 15: Keto Breakfast Recipes..**137**

  1. GLUTEN-FREE, KETO COCONUT BREAD 137

  2. BAKED BRUSSELS SPROUT WITH GARLIC 138

  3. SPINACH ROLLS...139

  4. LOW-CARB BREAKFAST BALLS..140

  5. KETO MUFFINS WITH CHICKEN 141

  6. BORECOLE WITH CURRY 142

  7. EGGS ON SOUR CREAM..143

  8. ZUCCHINI IN YOGURT 144

  9. GLUTEN-FREE, KETO COCONUT BREAD 145

  10. BAKED BRUSSELS SPROUT WITH GARLIC........................146

Chapter 16: Keto Smoothies **147**

  11. KETO GREEN SMOOTHIE..147

  12. KETO ALL IN ONE SMOOTHIE 148

  13. PUMPKIN PROTEIN SMOOTHIE 149

  14. GREEN PROTEIN SMOOTHIE 150

  15. HEALTHY GREEN SMOOTHIE...151

  16. SPINACH CUCUMBER SMOOTHIE...................................152

  17. SPINACH PEANUT BUTTER SMOOTHIE 153

  18. CHOCO FAT BOMB SMOOTHIE 154

  19. AVOCADO SMOOTHIE 155

  20. RASPBERRY SMOOTHIE...156

Chapter 17: Keto Snacks **157**

  21. SIMPLEST WRAPS EVER...157

  22. PEACHES AND CREAMY CHEESE 158

  23. THE HODGE PODGE GRAB BAG 159

  24. HEAVENLY MUSHROOMS...160

  25. SUNRISE KABOBS 161

  26. FISHY JERKY 162

  27. SAVORY WRAPS 163

  28. BEEF AND CHEESE 164

  29. TURKEY TUGS 165

  30. HARD BOILED POWER BALLS 166

Chapter 18: Keto Dressing, salads and Sauces....................................**167**

  31. PORK SALAD 167

  32. SALMON AND POTATO SALAD..169

33. CRISPY PORK SALAD...170
34. CAULIFLOWER TABOULE SALAD.............................172
35. CAPRESE SALAD..173
36. LOW-CARB MAYONNAISE FOR THE HORSERADISH DRESSING............175
37. VEGETARIAN CLUB SALAD...176
38. THAI PORK SALAD...178
39. EGG SALAD STUFFED AVOCADO...180
40. BISTRO STEAK SALAD WITH HORSERADISH DRESSING..................181

Chapter 19: Keto Fish Recipes....................................183
41. SHRIMP TUSCANY..183
42. SHRIMP IN TUSCAN CREAM SAUCE.....................................184
43. ALMOND PESTO SALMON..186
44. SALMON AND POTATO SALAD..187
45. CHILI LIME COD...188
46. MEDITERRANEAN TUNA..189
47. SMOKED SALMON..190
48. SALMON FISHCAKES...191
49. OMEGA-3 RICH SALMON SOUP...193
50. SPECIAL OCCASION'S CRAB LEGS......................................195

Chapter 20: Keto Meats recipes..................................197
51. BEEFY PIZZA...197
52. BACON CHEESEBURGER CASSEROLE....................................198
53. PAN-FRIED CHOPS...200
54. BALSAMIC BEEF ROAST..201
55. BACON & BBQ CHEESEBURGER WAFFLES............................203
56. CUMIN SPICED BEEF WRAPS...205
57. GROUND BEEF STIR FRY...206
58. CHICKEN FRIED PORK CHOPS..207
59. PARMESAN CRUSTED PORK CHOPS.....................................208
60. BEEF BURRITOS...209

Chapter 21: Keto Desserts...211
61. MINI CHOCOLATE CAKES..211
63. RICOTTA LEMON CHEESECAKE..212
64. WHEAT BELLY YOGURT..213
65. EGGS IN A CUP...214
66. VANILLA BEAN CHEESECAKE..215
70. PUMPKIN PECAN CAKE..216
71. CHOCOLATE CREAM...217

72. BUTTER PANCAKES 219
73. RASPBERRY COOKIES 220
74. VANILLA MOUSSE WITH CHOCOLATE SAUCE 222
75. SWEET ALMOND BUNS 223
76. COCOA PATTIES 225
77. EASY ALMOND BARS 226
78. PUMPKIN PIE PANCAKES 228
79. COCONUT BROWNIES WITH RASPBERRIES 229
80. CHOCOLATE CHIP COOKIES 231

Conclusion...**233**

INTRODUCTION

Thank you for purchasing this book. Living a keto lifestyle is possible for you, as long as you know about the diet and what you can and cannot eat. Ketogenic diet has revived the hope of individuals who are on the verge of giving up on their weight loss routine. This type of diet is quite unique, in the sense that it works on low carb diet composition; however, it does not put you in a starving mode, because you will simply replace most of the carbs with fat, vitamins and some proteins

The main reason why you find it difficult to lose weight is that your body has been conditioned to rely on carbs for energy. Carbs can be difficult to break down in the body system, and the fact that they slow down your metabolism simply means your weight loss will be ridiculously slow.

The Ketogenic weight loss diet works on a simple rule, and that is, to switch your body from carbohydrate-reliant to fat-burning mode. When your body enters ketosis, it uses up fat instead of carbs, and that means your body will burn fat faster than when it is on carb-burning mode. This book has comprehensive information about the ketogenic diet that will supercharge your weight loss journey.

Happy Reading!

CHAPTER 1: INTRODUCTION TO THE KETOGENIC DIET

What is the Ketogenic Diet?

The ketogenic or the keto diet for short is a well-known diet that has become popular because of the results it produces! It's a diet that is low in carbohydrates to induce the body into a state called ketosis. That is when the body's liver produces ketones to be used as energy instead of glucose that is produced when the body is on a normal carbohydrates diet. When you eat something that is high in carbohydrates, the body breaks down the sustenance to produce glucose and insulin. Glucose is the easiest molecule that the body stores energy in. Insulin processes the glucose in the bloodstream and takes it around the body. Because the body is making enough glucose to power you throughout the day, your fat molecules are not being used. By lowering the amount of carbohydrates, you are urging into a natural state of ketosis so it begins to burn fat instead. The ketones that the body produces are made from the breakdown of fats by the liver.

The ketones produced in your liver will be used for providing energy to your body. The carbohydrate intake is reduced drastically and replaced with fat. This forces your body to go into a state of ketosis. In turn, your body becomes much more efficient at burning fat and using it for energy instead of depending on carbohydrates. The fat in the liver is also converted to ketones which supply the brain with energy.

This forces the fat to get stored and makes you gain weight. However, now that you reduce the intake of carbohydrates, your body is forced to undergo ketosis. It is a natural mechanism of the body wherein the fats in the liver are broken down to produce ketones. This metabolic state is what helps you use the stored fat in your body as the main source of energy now.

There are different variants of the keto diet that you can follow:

- The standard ketogenic diet has very low carbohydrates, moderate protein content and high amount of fat. The high protein ketogenic diet has a higher amount of proteins than the standard diet.
- The targeted ketogenic diet involves adding carbohydrates in your diet according to your workout schedule.
- The cyclical ketogenic diet has a cycle where you follow a ketogenic diet for a certain number of days and then add carbs for a couple of days before switching back.

The Keto Diet is very low-carb. It's called the Ketogenic Diet because it's specifically designed to result in ketosis. What's ketosis? It sounds like a harmful disease that your body should be avoiding!

Nope, this isn't a harmful disease or state for your body to be in. Ketosis means that your liver, which is one of the most vital organs in your body, will start producing ketones. Those ketones will be like the liver is processing extra energy for you!

What happens if you stay on a diet that includes plenty of carbs? Every time you eat the bread, pasta, or flour biscuit, then your body is producing both glucose and insulin. Yes, every time you eat these foods, your body reacts by producing these small sugar molecules called glucose.

The Ketogenic Diet is a diet high in fat and low in carbohydrates, with an adequate amount of protein.

However, when you greatly reduce your intake of carbs—including while you're fasting or sleeping—your body loses its normal source of energy, carbs. This signals your body to start unlocking the fat stored in the body, and your liver starts converting this fat into ketone bodies, which pour into your bloodstream to replace glucose as your body's primary source of energy. As these ketones rush in to replace the glucose, your bloodstream is said to be in a state of "ketosis."

The Keto Diet encourages the eating of natural foods, as opposed to some of the other diets out there that push a bunch of processed powders full of artificial ingredients at you. So you can remain on the Keto Diet for the rest of your life. And it can change your life forever.

There's a certain flexibility in the diet to allow for differences in people and their needs, so the exact ratios of fats to carbs and proteins can vary slightly from person-to-person.

You could basically say that there are four basic types of Keto Diets, standard, high-protein, targeted and cyclical. The first two have been studied extensively and have been used by many people. The last two (cyclical and targeted) have not been studied extensively and are basically intended for athletes and body-builders. We don't recommend the last two diets at all for most people. Athletes and body-builders should only use them under the supervision of a person trainer, if at all.

And remember, when you're counting carbs, you need to subtract the grams of fiber from the total grams of carbs.

That glucose is then used as energy for your body. Maybe after you have your morning toast, you take a walk. Your body is using that glucose energy as you walk. This sounds like a good thing, right?

Well, not exactly. You see, glucose is being used as the primary energy. But, what about the fat in your body? When is that going to get used? When are you going to start burning fat? That's really what's going to make a difference in your weight loss goals!

You don't want to use the energy you just ate ten minutes ago. You want to use the stored fat on your body on your morning walk, so that you lose the weight. That's not going to happen on an eating plan that includes plenty of carbs.

But it will be on the Ketogenic Diet!

You don't want glucose energy from carbs to be used on your morning walk. You want the ketones from your liver. Ketones come from the breakdown of fats in the liver.

Your liver is going to be your best friend on the Keto Diet! Your liver processes every single thing that you eat. You want your liver to break down the fats you're eating and process those. Out come ketones, which are ready for you to use as energy on your morning walk.

It's kind of like switching from eating a cinnamon bun for breakfast to a carb-free energy bar. Sure, both of them technically 'feed' you calories that you can then use for energy. That's definitely true. But, which one is going to be processed by your body better? Which one is going to help you lose weight?

That's right – the energy bar. Without those carbs coming in, you're not feeding your body glucose. You're giving it other nutrients like fats and protein. That kicks your liver into producing ketones, and that is used as energy instead by your body.

How ketogenic diet is different from other low-carb diets

On the ketogenic diet, the optimal range for ketosis is anywhere between .5 and 3.0 mmol of ketones in your blood levels. If your blood levels are under, you are not in ketosis, and if they are over, then you are either entering starvation or are at risk of ketoacidosis. For now, however, focus on the optimal ketone zone which you will want to keep yourself in.

The ketogenic diet is more than just restricting your carbohydrates. However, the stricter you are with your carbs, the more likely you will be able to enter this state of ketosis. What is important to realize is that it will take more than lowering your carb intake to switch your body to ketones.

The ketogenic diet stands apart from other diets because it is a lifestyle change to a constant state of ketosis. Other diets such as the Atkin's diet and Paleo diet overlap in some areas, but fail to maintain the critical state of ketosis that allows for fat loss that is maintained.

The Atkin's diet calls for entering into a state of ketosis until a certain point at which you start reintroducing carbohydrates to your diet. The Atkin's diet is strictly a weight loss diet and not a way to keep the weight off. It is a quick fix that doesn't last. It uses some of the same principles as the ketogenic diet, but is intended to be temporary.

The Paleo diet is not strictly a low carbohydrate diet, but is often compared to the ketogenic diet. It focuses on eating whole foods that have not been processed down and were only available to our ancient ancestors. While it can induce a state of ketosis, it is not intended to. There are carbohydrates that are considered "good carbs" according to this plan. For example, sweet potatoes are considered good carbs on the Paleo diet. The problem with this is that you never sustain a state of ketosis, if you ever enter it, on the Paleo diet. This reduces the Paleo diets ability to consistently burn fat.

Keto Diet's History

In 1921, researcher Rollin Woodyatt found that the body produced three water-soluble compounds—collectively known as ketone bodies—when a person fasted or went on a low-carbohydrate diet. Because fasting had proven effective in the treatment of epilepsy, the medical establishment experimented with using the Keto Diet to treat epilepsy.

Not only did the Keto Diet prove effective in treating epilepsy, but epileptic patients could remain on the diet on a long-term basis without the obvious drawbacks and complications of fasting. So the medical establishment approved the diet for the treatment of epilepsy.

Pediatrician Mynie Peterman formulated the classic Keto Diet, and in 1925 reported that the diet had proven effective in reducing epileptic seizures in 95% of the thirty-seven patients she'd tested, with 60% of them becoming seizure-free.

The diet gained great popularity in the treatment of epilepsy in the 1920s and 1930s, until new anticonvulsive drugs were developed to treat epilepsy. The diet declined in use after than, mainly being confined to usage by the 25% of patients for whom the anticonvulsive drugs proved to be ineffective.

In the 1960s, people began using the Keto Diet for weight loss, but for the most part, the diet continued to toil in relative obscurity. That began to change in the 1990's, with TV exposure about how the diet had cured two cases of epileptic children where pharmaceutical treatment had failed. The first case was aired in 1994 on NBC's Dateline, concerning the son of Hollywood producer Jim Abrahams. The second case was aired in 1997, in a true-to-life movie entitled First Do No Harm, starring Meryl Streep.

What is Ketosis?

The good news is that many people are able to lose weight this way. On the other hand, some people find it difficult to enter this state and maintain a lifestyle with ketosis.

The word "keto" comes from the word "ketones" which are small molecules that the body is able to use as fuel. These are produced when your blood sugar becomes lower in supply. You are able to lower your blood sugar by eating fewer carbohydrates, higher fat concentrations, and a moderate amount of protein. These ketones (fuel) are produced in the liver from the fats you will be eating on this diet. However, the brain is not able to function off fat alone. This is why your body converts these fats into ketones.

Today, there is a belief that your brain needs carbohydrates to function properly, however, scientific studies have shown that this isn't necessarily true. In fact, studies have shown that your brain can work just as well on ketones as it does with your current diet, if not better while on the ketogenic diet as exampled by many people on the ketogenic diet reporting they have more focus and energy running off ketones compared to other diets.

Adaptation Steps of Our Body to Ketosis

So, it's going to take you at least one to two weeks to make the change to the Keto Diet. You're going to be adapting to a carb-less diet, and so is your body. Your whole life, you've been running your body mainly on carbs, so it's going to take some time to adapt.

What about carb cravings?

However, once you have made the switch, you'll definitely feel better. Also, because this diet stabilizes your blood sugar, it also stabilizes your energy.

The first phase - (about 8 hours from the last intake of carbohydrates).

The body still uses glucose, which came with the last intake of carbohydrates, but after 10 hours about 50% of the energy begins to come from the splitting of fatty acids.

The second phase - (1-2 days in the lack of carbohydrates.)

The body receives energy from cleavage fatty acids and liver glycogen (usually liver glycogen is consumed after 12-16 hours from the last intake of carbohydrates).

The third phase - (lasts for a week).

The body receives energy from the cleavage of fatty acids, and glucose, formed by gluconeogenesis from protein, lactate, pyruvate and glycerol. In this phase, there is a high probability of increased use of protein for gluconeogenesis.

The fourth phase - (comes in 5-7 days approximately).

This is almost a full adaptation of the body and entrance to ketosis.

In this phase, the decay of intrinsic protein and protein that comes with food slows down, and the brain already receives about 75% of the fuel it needs from ketones.

Now we know that the fewer carbohydrates and the longer they are gone - the closer our organism to ketosis. This is very important to understand. Even a very small amount of carbohydrates in the early days will withdraw your body from ketosis.

Therefore, it is important not to deceive yourself and not eat sweets, no matter how much you like it. Let's clarify the answer to the question, exciting many active people and myself including.

What about the carbohydrates before the training?

Maybe, a limited number should be taken?

Types of Ketosis

There are a couple of ways to enter ketosis besides the popular practice of lowering your carb intake and consuming foods that are higher in fat. This specific type of ketosis is known as nutritional ketosis. Below, we will outline several other ways of entering ketosis if you feel the more popular way doesn't fit your lifestyle.

Carbohydrate-Restricted Ketosis

This is one of three variations of nutritional ketosis, and one of the most popular. Diet is very important in this version of ketosis; however, the macronutrient distribution can change drastically in individuals. When on a high fat and low carb diet, there is an increase in fat oxidation, so this diet is best for those who are looking for a sustainable, long-term approach to the ketogenic diet.

11

Supplemental Ketosis

For some of the benefits that come with the ketogenic diet, it will take a bit more than restricting your carb intake for this diet to be effective. This is especially true at the levels of ketones that can be a bit difficult to maintain while on the ketogenic diet. For those who have trouble keeping their levels steady, there are supplements for this. As mentioned earlier, there are supplements known as MCTs which help you to maintain and increase ketone levels for a longer period of time. If you have chronic health issues and are attempting to cure them with a change in your diet, you will want to consider this version of the ketogenic diet.

Fasting Ketosis

Ketosis occurs when blood glucose and insulin levels drop in your body at which point the fat oxidation begins to increase, allowing your body to produce the ketones. At first, this will only be about .1 mmol/L to .3 mmol/L. As you continue to fast, the number of ketones will increase. If you are looking for a jumpstart way to enter ketosis, this is the best option for you.

Signs You are in Ketosis

There are several symptoms that you may experience, so we suggest going to the doctor's office to officially test if you are in a state of ketosis. However, if you choose to skip going to the doctor, there are several signs of ketosis you can detect by yourself. Keep a close eye out for the following signs to assure you are in a state of ketosis:

Dry Mouth

As your body enters ketosis, you may find your mouth becoming drier than usual or that you feel thirstier. Ultimately, you will want to be sure that you are well hydrated while on the ketogenic diet.

Increased Urination

As you drink more liquids, you will also notice an increased need to urinate. Additionally, acetoacetate, one of the ketone bodies, is able to build up in your urine. You can take an at-home urine test to determine the number of acetoacetates in your urine.

Ketone Scent

One of the more popular symptoms of the ketogenic diet is the ketogenic smell. For many people, this is what is known as "ketone breath", but it can also be produced via sweat. For some, this scent is fruity, but for others, it can smell like nail polish remover.

Loss of Hunger

For those looking to lose weight, this may be an exciting symptom for you to experience. Many people on the ketogenic diet experience a reduced appetite which is mostly due to the way that the body burns energy by using fat storage while in ketosis. Some people have even reported eating one or two meals a day while on the ketogenic diet and still feeling satisfied.

How to Measure Ketones

Measuring your ketone level is going to be vital during this diet. It is important that you keep your body in a state of ketosis so that you don't have to keep fasting to get back into it.

Judging from Symptoms of Ketosis

This doesn't cost money, but it isn't as reliable as the other methods, nor does it give you the exact levels of ketones. The normal symptoms that your body is entering ketosis can vary from person-to-person, but here are the most common: (1). Increased urination.

(2). Dry mouth and increased thirst. It's okay to counter this by drinking more water. You can also add salt to your diet, unless salt causes you issues or you have problems with high blood pressure.

(3). Acetone breath. Acetone is a ketone that can be excreted through the breath; it has a fruity smell. This symptom is normally temporary.

(4). Increased energy. You might experience a temporary decline in energy when you first go onto the diet as your body adjusts to the change. But oftentimes, once your body makes the adjustment to the diet and enters ketosis, you'll experience higher levels of energy.

(5) Reduced hunger. Because fat is a steadier and more reliable source of energy than glucose, once you start entering ketosis, you're apt to experience fewer and milder hunger pangs.

Urine Strips

Urine strips are the easiest and cheapest way to definitely determine whether you've entered ketosis, though you won't know the exact ketone levels. You can buy these strips online or from any drug store. The instructions can vary from brand to brand, but normally you just pee in a cup and dip the strip into it for about fifteen seconds. The strip will turn a different color if you're in ketosis, as per the instructions. For many people, this is the cheapest and easiest way to measure your ketones. If you are just beginning the ketogenic diet, this may be the best option for you as you simply have to stick the strip into a cup of your fresh urine. The strip's color will then change depending on the level of ketones that are in your system in that moment. If the strip turns a dark purple color, you will know that you are indeed in a state of ketosis.

One problem with urine strips is that they only are completely reliable for at most a few weeks, because your body then becomes more efficient at reabsorbing ketones from urine, so you won't be losing as many ketones to your urine. So you should make sure you use the urine strips daily from the beginning of your diet and continue using them after you start getting positive results. And then, if you start getting negative results, you can switch to a different method for monitoring your ketone level.

Breath Analyzer.

These instruments determine ketosis levels from your breath. Like urine strips, they give you a color code for a general ketone level rather than an exact measurement, and they aren't always completely reliable. You can get them for about $150 online or in drug stores. The breath analyzer is a device that is able to measure the amount of ketones on your breath, so this may be a good device for you to check your body's ketosis level if you are short on time. The good news is that this device is both simple and reusable, unlike urine strips; however, it may not always be reliable. This is because the number of ketones on your breath can change depending on the time of day, and may even change from breath to breath. If you do not need an exact number, this still may be a good option for you!

Blood Ketone Meter.

These babies measure ketone levels exactly and are much more reliable than the other three choices. They're similar to the test diabetics use for testing their blood sugar. You prick the side of your finger to get a drop of blood and then put the drop on a strip for a machine to measure. It's usually an easy and straightforward process. Just follow the instructions and dispose of the needles properly. These meters cost about $100 and include several strips.

If you are not queasy at the sight of blood, the ketone meter blood test may be a good option for you. This is the most reliable method currently available, but the device itself tends to be fairly expensive. Additionally, if you have a low pain tolerance, this will not be a feasible option as you will need to prick your finger for each test.

How to enter ketosis

Let most of your fat calories come from the healthy kinds alternatives, particularly monounsaturated fats, saturated fats and omega 3s.

If your net carb limit is low, you should avoid fruits and other low-carb treats.

Don't starve yourself. Ensure that you eat whenever you are hungry.

While it helps to keep an eye on your calorie intake, you should never ignore your body's needs. Drink at least 2-3 liters of water daily.

Stock up on healthy foods like non-starchy vegetables, meat, eggs, coconut oil, avocado, macadamia nuts, bone broth and other fermented foods, saturated fats, and unsaturated fats.

Avoid processed fats like vegetable oils, fully and partially hydrogenated oils, margarine, trans fats, soybean oil, corn oil and canola oil.

Raw and organic dairy products are also good as long as you don't have any allergies. However, you should try to avoid milk due to its high carb content or opt for unpasteurized full-fat milk if you have to.

Increase your electrolyte intake. The ketogenic diet may cause sodium, calcium and potassium deficiencies, so you should increase your intake of mushrooms, salmon and avocados for potassium; nuts or magnesium supplements for magnesium; and salt or bone broth for sodium.

Avoid processed foods as these tend to contain hidden carbs such as sorbitol, maltitol, preservatives, additives and artificial sweeteners. To be on the safe side, be sure to always read the labels when shopping.

If you are using any medications that contain sugars or sweeteners, ask for the sugar-free variety. Make sure you always plan your diet in advance to avoid temptation and spontaneous eating.

Shop weekly and get rid of anything that is not allowed on the diet from your home. Have salads and hard boiled eggs available in case you feel like snacking.

Let us now get to the specifics; what should you eat and what should you avoid while on a ketogenic diet in order to get into a state of ketosis effortlessly? Let's start with what to eat.

CHAPTER 2: HOW METABOLISM WORKS WHEN YOU ARE ON THE KETOGENIC DIET

Metabolism is a complex process which describes how the body breaks down the food we eat into energy for all our living processes. Often, people will blame their metabolism for not being able to lose weight, but the truth is, there are many other factors involved. Your age, sex, and body size all play a role in your metabolic rate. Those differences are normal and are not usually the cause of weight gain.

Many diets try and limit your caloric intake as if that will increase your metabolic rate. But it does the opposite! When you're depriving your body of food and limiting your daily intake, your body begins to store every single calorie in what you do eat. You want to spread out your meals during the day and eat a healthy diet instead of staying hungry all day or only eating one giant meal.

It can be harder to maintain weight loss if you were overweight before. Researchers aren't sure of the exact science behind this, but it's theorized that hormonal changes that occur after you lose weight can slow your metabolism and make you feel hungrier. Sometimes you can get medication to help with this sensation, but it's important that you're aware of your caloric intake so you are not overeating and regaining the weight.

The real problem occurs when you're eating more calories than you're consuming. That leaves your body with excess food intake that it stores as fat. The best way to lose weight is to have a balance of a healthy diet and staying active. That way, you are aware of how much you are eating and what types of food you are ingesting, and you are burning off any excess energy with exercise.

The keto diet capitalizes on eating the right foods to give you a fulfilled sensation. By eating healthier fats and protein, the body is burning from the fat reserves it has stored, instead of producing new molecules. With the right meal plan and a combination of steady exercise, the keto diet can produce weight loss and reduce the amount of insulin secreted.

Metabolic Effects of the Ketogenic Diet

One topic that always raises controversy whenever the ketogenic diet comes under the spotlight is whether the diet can mess up your metabolism.

Basically, the main purpose of your metabolic system is to make fuels available in your body whenever they are needed. As you continue on with the diet, your metabolic system continues to work to ensure that the energy from the foods you eat is appropriately allocated and the excess stored. The average human today eats much more than is recommended, and as a result the metabolic system has to cope with more work than it is designed to handle.

During a starvation diet, your metabolic system concentrates on providing glucose to tissues that need it to function, for instance, the brain, kidney, red blood cells, etc.

This glucose is usually obtained from your body's protein stores; mainly the muscles and sometimes fat. As your body continues to utilize proteins from the muscles for energy, your muscle mass begins to decrease, leaving your metabolic system with two challenges; how to continue supplying glucose to the glucose-dependent tissues, and how to maintain muscle mass so that your body doesn't become too weak to function.

Your metabolic system doesn't know how long this starvation will last, it could be a few hours or a couple of weeks. It first tries to cope by plundering the glucose supply in your blood, before proceeding to the proteins in your muscles. But because it must also ensure that your muscle mass is not excessively depleted, it is forced to turn to the ketones for energy.

Ketones stand in for glucose and proteins, sparing your muscles from being depleted. This is what happens on a starvation diet.

On a typical low-carb diet, you would need to consume some proteins and fats in order to preserve your muscles. The proteins you consume are converted to glucose. The question is, will a low-carb diet ruin your metabolism?

Macronutrients Break Down

Once you decide which version of the ketogenic diet that you will adopt, it will be important to learn how to track and follow your macronutrients as these factors will be important when you are building your plate on the ketogenic diet. The three macronutrients include carbs, protein, and fats. If you choose the standard ketogenic diet as traditionally recommended, your diet will be low carb, moderate protein, and high fat. While these macronutrient numbers will vary depending on your own individual goals, you can get the gist of the plan based on the general range.

Carb Intake

As a general rule, you will be eating anywhere from twenty to fifty grams of carbohydrates every day totaling to roughly five to ten percent of your total calories. As mentioned above, this number can range. For example, some individuals are able to consume one hundred grams of carbohydrates a day and still remain in ketosis while others can only consume twenty or thirty. Regardless, you will need to learn your body and follow the rules accordingly.

Protein Intake

Your protein intake will be a vital component of your diet. Protein will help you prevent injury, will help to promote longevity, and can also help to maintain muscle mass. You can determine your protein consumption by calculating your activity level and body composition. For most people, you will need anywhere from .7 to .0 grams of protein per lean body mass pound. For example, if you are a female and weigh 150 pounds, you can expect to consume anywhere from 105 to 135 grams of protein per day.

Fat Intake

Once you have calculated the number of carbohydrates and amount of protein you need every day, you will subtract this number from 100. When you have this number, this is the percentage of calories you will need to consume via fat. For example, if your diet is 20% protein and 5% carbohydrate, you will need to get the remaining 75% of calories from fat.

Ultimately, there will be no need to count calories while on the ketogenic diet. Instead, you will need to focus on your macro levels. One of the easier ways to do this is to use a **keto macro calculator**. For some people, reaching ketosis is easier than others, but this will all be based around factors including gender, age, body composition, lifestyle, and activity level. By using a calculator, you will be able to determine your macro levels necessary to keep your body in ketosis.

Fats and Carbs in the Keto Diet

The keto diet's goal is to limit the amount of carbohydrates consumed and to eat healthy fats to quench your hunger and meet the macronutrient requirements of your body. Macronutrients are the body's energy building blocks of carbs, fats, and proteins. By limiting the amount of carbs, you want to meet your macro intake by increasing the amount of the other two groups to fulfill your hunger. Every person has their individual ratio of macronutrients. Most people have a standard diet of about 50% carbohydrates, 30% protein, and 20% fats. What the keto diet does is change the ratio of these nutrients. By limiting the amount of carbs and increasing the intake of the other two groups, the body goes into the natural state of ketosis and begins to burn ketones that it creates from the fat molecules you have stored.

What most people on a keto diet do is try and restrict their carb intake to less than 50 grams of net carbs a day. If you have 20 grams of carbs but 5 grams of that is fiber, then you have eaten 15 net carbs from that food item. Carbohydrates include items like bread, beans, pasta, rice, and sugar. You want to compensate for the loss of those food groups by incorporating more protein into your diet and filling up with healthy snacks like nuts.

Fats will consist of the majority of your diet on a keto plan, so you want to make your meal choices with your favorite snacks in mind. You can also add fat to your meals in the form of a salad dressing mixed with olive oil, or just adding a slice of grass-fed butter on top of your meat. Even when cooking, try and use healthy oils like coconut oil, avocado oil, or ghee which is a great way to up your fat servings.

Carbohydrate Loading

Carbohydrate loading is used for cyclic keto diets, which are perhaps the most popular variant of this diet.

The essence of carbohydrate loading is that you deplete carbohydrate stores for a week, and then during the day, you eat carbohydrates, "pulling" the body from the state of ketosis and spurring metabolism. If we say quite accurately, it means to spur production of row enzymes, and especially the hormone of adipose tissue - leptin, which is necessary for normal fat burning.

During the phase of glycogen depletion, you generally do not eat foods containing carbohydrates.

No fruit, sweets, bread, cookies, ketchup, cereals, pasta, potatoes, etc.

All this is completely prohibited.

Do not be lazy to check what is written on the packaging in order to make sure of the absence of carbohydrates. Acceptable consumption of 20-50 gr. fiber (fibrous carbohydrates, vegetables) per day.

It can be green vegetables without additives, in which most often there are simple carbohydrates. At one meal, not more than 5-10 grams of such vegetables is permissible.

Less is better, than more!

If you are not sure about the absence of carbohydrates, then do not eat the dish.

Remember that the more active you are, the more you train (especially with iron), the faster your stores of glycogen (carbohydrate) deplete.

For example, if you have three workouts per week, then you may need a week to enter the 4th phase (ketosis), and if you have at least one workout every day, then on the 3rd or 4th day you can enter into active ketosis (phase 4).

The rule is very simple: the deeper depletion of energy, the faster switching to fat! However, only when there are no carbohydrates in the system.

Carbohydrate loading is permissible only when you have reached ketosis and at least a couple of days stayed in it actively burning fat.

This is a very important moment.

The first time you can stay without carbohydrates for two weeks, and subsequent loadings conduct once a week.

How long does carbohydrate load last?

Most often recommend from half to one and a half days (12-36 hours).

My opinion is a maximum 12 hours!!!

And most often even less (9 hours).

For example, if you woke up at 9.00 and ate carbohydrates, then the last carbohydrate intake is acceptable around 18.00 pm.

In this interval, you can use any carbohydrates (simple and complex, except fruit and ice cream) with each meal for the amount of 50-100 gr.

The exact figure for carbohydrates per day = 10 grams of carbohydrates per kg of dry body weight (dry body weight = weight without fat).

In humans, the amount of fat on average is 15-20% of the total body weight, but in general, it is an individual indicator, depending on the characteristics of the structure.

The intake of proteins can be kept high during the loading phase, but the intake of fats should be reduced as a balance to receive more carbohydrates.

In essence: you need to replenish muscle glycogen stores for intensive training next week. This is necessary for better muscle maintenance and increasing level of leptin. Hence the remark: if for you your muscle is not important, and the main priority is fat burning, then you can minimize the load, or even completely abandon it for a long time (constant keto diet).

Why can't you eat fruit and ice cream?

Because fructose and lactose are easily deposited as glycogen in the liver (not in muscles, like other carbohydrates).\

This will slow the entry into ketosis during depletion next week because you will spend "extra stock" before fat begins to burn.

Fructose is a simple (fast) sugar found in any sweet fruit, and lactose is a simple milk sugar found in milk-based products. This does not mean that you cannot eat an apple or drink a milkshake but it means that it is wiser to give preference to a piece of cake than fruit and ice cream. By the way, now you understand why sportsmen on a diet intuitively exclude milk.

One of the reasons is a slowdown in fat burning.

How to Balance Your Hormones on a Keto Diet?

There is some misinformation out there that states that the keto diet can cause a hormone imbalance. But most of the research states that the keto diet is a great way to balance your hormone levels and especially to regulate your insulin levels. Insulin is produced by the pancreas in response to the body processing carbohydrates and creating glucose molecules. In most diets, an excess amount of carbs will increase your blood sugar and can result in insulin resistance. But the great news is that a keto diet minimizes your carbohydrates intake. This is successful at regulating your blood sugar better and maintaining normal insulin production. This greatly reduces your risk of diabetes. Cortisol is the stress hormone we mentioned earlier. When the body has a high carbohydrate intake, blood sugar rises quickly then drops due to the food intake. Because of this chemical reaction, the body produces cortisol in response to the stress. Thanks to the ketogenic diet, the body is shown to regulate blood sugar much better, which reduces the stressful spikes in blood sugar, which means less cortisol production. This takes the stress off your adrenal glands so they produce the stress hormone at the appropriate times, leading to the correct hormone balance in your body.

PCOS, or Polycystic Ovary Syndrome, occurs in women who have an imbalance in their reproductive hormones. It's the most common cause of infertility in women and it can be heartbreaking to live with when couples are trying to conceive. Though there is no cure to PCOS, the keto diet has become a popular method to try and treat the symptoms involved in PCOS. Things like high blood glucose levels, insulin resistance, and obesity are associated with PCOS. Studies have shown that women who started the keto diet have shown remarkable improvements in those areas and managed to regulate their insulin and hormone levels. This can lead to a better overall quality of life, reduce their risk of diseases, and has even contributed to a greater chance of a successful pregnancy. Leanne Vogel who runs a successful fitness and nutrition podcast that's ranked in the top 10 in the U.S. and Canada has attributed the keto diet to resolving her low hormone. The keto diet has even been shown to have a positive effect on reducing the symptoms of PMS that women can experience before their menstrual cycle. Things like a headache, irritability, mood swings, and acne. A healthy, clean ketogenic diet can ease those symptoms and regulate a woman's hormone levels at this time of the month.

Ketones are also a great way to regulate your immune system. This can be the key to healing your other organs that could be involved in other diseases. For example, some diseases can occur where your glands become overactive, like hypothyroidism or autoimmune diseases where the body's organs turn on itself. With autoimmune diseases, in particular, it's not the organ's fault but it's the immune system that's incorrectly seeing it as an invader and attacking it. Ketone production is a great way to heal your immune system which can mean eventually healing the organs involved in hormone imbalance.

The way that the keto diet regulates hormones is by being a diet of high-quality fats and proteins. Hormones are composed of lipids (the scientific term for fat molecules), amino acids (protein molecules), and cholesterol. Sex hormones, in particular, are created by cholesterol and saturated fat. The ketogenic involves eating a high-quality diet of all of the above nutrients! So, it makes perfect sense to see how scientifically this diet can regulate your hormone levels and create healthy new hormones in your body.

Think of it this way - the keto diet is set up to allow your body to naturally form ketones to use as energy. This is the same action the body would take if there were no carbohydrates to consume. Keto followers are just voluntarily making the decision. The body is set up by evolution to adapt to its circumstances regarding sustenance. It naturally falls into the state of ketosis to use ketones as energy when there is a shortage of carbs and it cannot produce glucose. Due to this natural process, the body's hormone levels would adapt to the lack of carbohydrates as well. A keto diet capitalizes on those adjustments of the body to live an overall healthier lifestyle.

CHAPTER 3: KETOGENIC DIET AND WEIGHT LOSS

This is going to be an interesting portion that we are moving into. Weight loss! And more importantly how ketogenic diet will help to achieve that. We shall be having a brief on what exactly brings about weight loss, the more common principles for successful weight loss and also some useful, actionable tips at the end as well.

When your body finds itself in a state where calories input is lesser than what it needs to daily function, it will seek to get energy from stores of energy within your body. Most of the time these would be from the stores of glucose found in the liver as well as from your muscle. The other major energy store found in our body would be the fats that we carry on our frame. This is where the tricky part comes in. If your body isn't conditioned for burning fats, it will quickly use up the glucose stores, and that is when the feeling of hunger will come into potentially derail you from your weight loss mission.

Being mindful of hunger – As we said earlier, keeping hunger pangs at bay is one of the most important ways to ensure your weight loss regime is on track.

The other spiffy thing about going on the keto diet is the resultant leveling of your insulin levels. Insulin is known to induce the feeling of hunger and when ketosis kicks in, you no longer have those roller coaster ups and downs that are associated with the consumption of carbs and with that stability means your hunger pangs are held largely at bay due to the reduction of insulin produced by your body.

Now, you will eat when your body truly feels hunger, and that is quite liberating. Not to mention that because of this removal of hunger pangs from the overall equation, your weight loss journey will become much, much simpler.

Quicker recovery from exercise – While we engage in strength training in our bid to lose weight and get in shape, our bodies need time to recover from the physical activity. Practitioners of the keto diet will find that their recovery time will be somewhat quicker than others.

With the more stable energy levels achieved due to fewer fluctuations in the blood sugar levels, again due to the diet switch, this then allows you to work out without feeling faintish or light-headed, typical symptoms of hypoglycemia or just simple lack of glucose in the bloodstream. Because you are burning fats and producing ketones as a more stable energy source!

More motivation from quicker results – Quick question, which would you prefer, a weight loss method that requires you to toil consistently at it for up to six months a pop, and having a loss of four or five pounds to show for it, or ketogenic diet that can see weight loss come in the range of twenty to thirty pounds within six to seven weeks?

If you are like me, then the choice would be the latter. Quicker results, especially in the area of weight loss, is almost always going to be a welcome morale booster. When you see how much weight you have lost within those short weeks, it gives you that confidence that this method works and you gain that conviction and strength to keep going.

What happens here when you transit over to the keto diet is the fact that you have lowered insulin levels. Heightened insulin tells our kidneys to retain more salt and water, so when the insulin levels decrease, we have consequently lesser salt and water retention. This leads to a quick decrease in the number on the weighing scales, but more importantly, the keto diet also provides for a sustained drive in the loss of body weight through the burning of fat stores.

How do you lose weight on the Ketogenic Diet? It sounds like some kind of fantasy to expect that eating 70% fats and 19% proteins helps you lose weight.

But it does!

It also sounds too good to be true that you can start the Keto Diet no matter what age you are, no matter how much weight you have to lose, and no matter how many other diets or eating plans you've tried in the past.

However, this is also true!

The Keto Diet helps you not only achieve your weight loss goals, but it also gives your body a new kind of health that you've probably not experienced before.

How does Ketogenic diet help you lose weight?

What your body is designed to eat will definitely affect whether you lose weight or not. The earliest humans often rely on what they get during hunting to survive, these include; edible foods, fish and meat, with little or no starch or carb, and that is one of the reasons why they stay slimmer and healthier. With the discovery of processed foods in the modern world (including pasta, white bread and sugary drinks), our bodies have been re-constructed to adjust to such unhealthy lifestyles.

One problem with most starch and sugar is that they can be converted into simple sugars that can be absorbed readily in the blood stream, and the effect of this is that there is a rapid increase in blood sugar level, a condition that triggers a sharp increase in the secretion of Insulin hormones, and this increases the risk of developing diseases such as diabetes type II through rapid weight gain and obesity.

One problem with carbs and sugars is that they increase your cravings, while Ketogenic diet helps you feel fuller quickly and reduce them. The early men consume more of ketogenic diets, and that is why they consume much less but get more energy for hunting expenditures. Ketogenic diets help lower your body's reliance on insulin hormones, and then makes it easier for the body to use up its fat reservoir as a source of energy.

You don't have to starve yourself to enjoy the benefits of Ketogenic diet, likewise, there is no need to start counting those calories.

Some Common Weight Loss Principles to Note

Many people think that an all meat diet is very appealing but remember that the ketogenic diet does not work this way. It is important that you watch what you put into your plate so that your body can maintain ketosis. But while knowing how much fat, protein, and carbs is important, it is not enough to promote healthy weight loss. Thus, here are top tips on how to lose as much weight while following the ketogenic diet within the shortest possible time.

Weigh Your Food

Being accurate about your macros is very crucial to the success of the ketogenic diet. Make sure that invest in a good food scale so that you can monitor your macro intake. So, avoid the guesswork and use a scale to measure your food. If you have more money to spare, buy scales that you can connect to apps and websites.

To help with the process of losing the unwelcome weight from your body, here are some of the more common principles which are good to base your weight loss strategies on.

Keep hunger at bay

Many folks start off on dieting to lose their excess weight and attempt to get healthy, but quite a number fail and fall by the wayside. In the end, these folks have to resort to medications and drugs to suppress the symptoms and conditions that accompany obesity. It is not a pretty sight, and it sometimes is quite depressing to see people consign themselves to such a fate when more efficient and healthier solutions are just around the corner.

They may have started off strong and seen results after some time, but invariably, the one thing that always put paid to these efforts would be the feeling of hunger that many of these diets entail. Take a plain calorie restriction diet plan for example, if your daily requirement works out to be about 1,750 calories, just polishing off a bagel for a snack would set you back by 250 calories. That is like one-seventh of your total requirement. Imagine eating seven bagels for the whole day, would that be enough?

The trick, of course, is to get onto a diet and lifestyle change where you can feel full and keep the hunger pangs at bay and yet get your body to lose weight. Know of any diet that does just that?

Be sustainable

There are many ways to lose weight, that is for sure. Getting on the latest fad diet, juicing, fasting, going the vegan way.

Fasting, for example, is a good way to let the body rebalance itself and to get rid of toxins that have built up over time. One of the side effects of fasting would be a loss of body weight. However, you would not expect a person to fast for a lifetime, without any consumption of food. For any method of efficient weight loss, it must be sustainable in practice to allow for continued shedding of the excess pounds and also to prevent the dreaded bounce back in weight that has plagued so many.

One of the benchmarks of sustainability for diets would be the ease of implementing it in everyday life. Imagine if you are on a diet that requires you to eat six to seven small meals a day, you would have to pack for those meals and also find the time to consume them during the workday.

Exercise

Regarded as one of the main pillars for weight loss, exercise, especially strength training, can help to build muscles that burn more calories, not to mention getting you that ripped figure. Yes, it was always good to dream that there was some magic pill in the market that could get you whipped into shape without any effort, but alas, it remains a dream.

Strength training, done through weights at home or by hitting the gym is one of the surest ways that weight can be lost. Most of the time, it would be advisable to have a schedule for the days that your workout to concentrate on specific muscle groups. This targeted training helps to speed muscle development, leading to higher calorie usage and hence weight loss.

There will be loads of resources online on how to work out a proper strength training routine. The more important thing is to have the discipline to keep plugging at it until you see or feel the results. It will be worth it.

Reduce Your Stress

Stress can affect your hormone levels by causing your blood sugar level to rise thus increasing your cravings. Have you ever noticed why you often crave for sweets when you are stressed out? That's your hormone talking. While you cannot control the stress that comes your way, find ways on how to mitigate it. You can practice yoga, mindfulness, and breathing exercises to take away your stress.

Choose Quality Carbs

Some of you may say that carb is carb no matter what form they exist in. But remember that not all carbs are created equally. There are carbs that are nutrient-rich and are found in non-starchy vegetables and some fruits. So, when making a meal plan, make sure that you use good quality carbs.

Stay Away from Diet Soda

Just because it comes with the word "diet" with it does not mean that it is good for you. Diet soda uses a wide variety of sugar substitutes that tells your body that is has an overload of sugar thereby shutting the metabolism down. So, if you need to quench your thirst, drink sparkling water instead.

Get Enough Sleep

Sleep is necessary in order for you to lose weight fast. Remember that the lack of sleep causes stress to the body. Stress, as I have discussed earlier can affect the hormone levels in your body thus increasing your cravings to constantly snack on food. So, make sure that you get at least 6 to 8 hours of sleep daily.

Intermittent Fasting:

If you truly want to lose weight fast with the ketogenic diet, you might want to consider pairing it with intermittent fasting. Intermittent fasting is when you fast for more than 12 hours so that your body will use up the stored fats as its primary fuel. Consume your keto-friendly meals within a short eating window time and the rest of the day should be dedicated to no food consumption so that your body can undergo the state of ketosis faster.

Sports and Keto Diet?

What is healthier and more effective for getting rid of excess weight: the keto diet or intensive exercise in conjunction with the usual high-carbohydrate diet?

One group for 10 weeks followed the keto diet: its participants consumed no more than 30 grams of carbohydrates per day, without doing any physical exercise.

Participants in the second group followed the so-called "standard American diet", i.e. They ate the high-carbohydrate food habitual for themselves, also without doing any physical exercise.

And in the third group, participants ate ordinary high-carb foods, doing sports for 30 minutes 3-5 times a week.

Researchers measured a number of indicators of participants at the beginning and end of the research, incl. body mass index, triglyceride level in blood, a percentage of adipose tissues, glycated hemoglobin level (HgA1c) and ketone level in the blood.

Participants in the group following ketogenic low-carbohydrate diet were in diet ketosis - i.e. in a state where the main source of energy for the body is not glucose, but special molecules - ketones, produced by the liver from fat.

The results of analyzes showed that, as might be expected, sports or physical activities are useful but not enough to neutralize the negative consequences of malnutrition and reverse metabolic syndrome. However, following the ketogenic diet led to the most significant improvement in almost all indicators of metabolic health and weight loss.

In addition, the members of the keto group significantly increased the level of basal metabolism (speed) which the body "burns" fat at resting state - more than 10 times compared with two groups of "standard" nutrition.

Authors of the research stated, "Physiological ketosis has the clinical capabilities to prevent, weaken and heal the metabolic syndrome and the obesity, prediabetes and diabetes that it causes, and is therefore a worthy alternative treatment."

CHAPTER 4: CLARIFYING THE COMMON MYTHS ABOUT THE KETOGENIC DIET

Carbohydrates as an essential macronutrient

This is simply not true. It is a very old myth which hast no fundament, no real study to prove it. Essential, as a medical term, means that the human body can't synthesize the nutrient itself which means you have to get it through your diet. In case of carbohydrates we all learn as kids in school, that everything could be broke down in carbs if needed.

One very common saying is, that we need carbohydrates in order to produce the fuel for a healthy and good functioning brain. What these people don't know is, that this is only the case if you are going on a high carb diet which causes your brain to rely on more then usual amounts of carbohydrates. Our skeletal muscles burn fatty acids preferentially to spare glucose for the brain. However, once a person is keto-adapted "your brain switches to ketoburn-mode and uses ketone bodies for over half its energy needed.

If you look on people like the Inuit or the Masai of Africa, you will not see any health issues because of their nutrition. So how you can see, carbs are definitely not an essential nutrient for a healthy lifestyle.

Ketogenic diet is dangerous because of Ketosis

This is a Myth that will show you for sure that your opponent has just no clue about the term Ketogenic Diet. It's because they change up the terms ketosis and ketoacidosis.

Ketosis is just what happens to your body when you use a controlled Ketogenic Diet. Your insulin levels get regulated which results in production of fatty acids and ketones, caused either by a fast or a reduction in carbs.

Ketoacidosis is caused by a too low concentration of insulin in your body. Without it the blood sugar immediately rises which results in a stream of stored fat out of fat cells. Because of this your body starts to produce high amounts of ketones which interferences in combination with high blood sugar the normal acid/base-balance of the system to a stage it can be very dangerous.

And this is with Ketosis surely not the case. So it is just another myth that is causes by a lack of knowledge.

There will be tremendous damage for your kidneys because of high Protein consumption

Just like the Myths mentioned above, this one is based on a lack of knowledge. Nobody ever said, that the Ketogenic Diet (or any other diet based on low carb) is low in carbohydrates and instead high in protein.

So no — your kidney will surely not be damaged because of a high consumption of proteins, it is just not the case.

The ketogenic diet is just a fad diet

The ketogenic diet cannot be truthfully labeled as a fad diet. Anyone who says it is a fad diet is either ignorant of the facts or is probably trying to sell you something. As we have already seen, the ketogenic diet has been recognized for almost 100 years as a treatment for epilepsy. But going back even further, we see that low carbohydrate diets are even older still. The first low carbohydrate diet was published in 1863. At that time it saw great success too.

In addition to being such an old concept for dieting, low carbohydrate diets have been proven to work in more than 22 different scientific studies just since 2003. So we are talking about a fad that has been around more than 150 years and has a proven track record of success for people. In fact, that doesn't really sound like a fad diet at all. Fad diets may come and go every year, but the ketogenic diet is not one of them. It has been around a long time and will continue to be a successful way for people to lose weight for a long time to come.

The ketogenic diet is hard to stick to

Some say that the ketogenic diet is harder than other diets to stick to because you have to remove entire food groups from your diet. This causes a person to crave the missing food groups and they ultimately end up breaking their diet as a result. All diets cut something out though, whether that is a food group or calories. The problem with the idea that ketogenic dieting is harder to stick to, however, is that you can actually eat until you are full. People who restrict calories on the other hand do not get the luxury of ever being satisfied with a meal. That is a definite recipe for breaking your diet.

The ketogenic diet will ruin your physical performance

Many people believe that carbohydrates are essential for peak physical performance. The majority of top athletes eat a high carbohydrate diet so it follows that it must be the best diet to perform your best. It is true that your physical performance will suffer in the beginning of the ketogenic diet. This is because your body is adapting to using fat for energy. However, after you give yourself a few weeks to get used to the new changes, you will find that the ketogenic diet no longer inhibits you. Several studies have confirmed that low carbohydrate diets like the ketogenic diet improve physical performance in the long term, especially endurance activities. One such study published in 2014 in the British Journal of Sports Medicine found that as long as people are given a few weeks to adapt, they perform better while on the low carbohydrate diet. Other studies, including one published in 2014 in the Journal of the International Society of Sports Medicine, have found the low carbohydrate dieting is beneficial to muscle strength and mass.

Ketosis is a damaging metabolic state

This idea is a confusion of two different metabolic terms. Ketosis is often confused with ketoacidosis. Ketosis is when your body synthesizes ketones from fat for fuel. Ketoacidosis is a dangerous condition that is typically caused by uncontrolled type I diabetes. Ketoacidosis is when the blood stream is flooded with ketones to the point where it turns acidic. It can be fatal if it is not treated. You will never enter a state of ketoacidosis while on the ketogenic diet. Something has to be wrong with your body for ketoacidosis to occur.

Low Carb intake causes muscles to shrink

Clearly the opposite is the case. There a several studies showing us, that people who went on a calorie deficit with high carb low fat nutrition lost more pure muscle mass then people who did the same just with a low carb high fat nutrition. The main factor for keeping the amount of muscle mass up is for sure a high enough intake of proteins which you will definitely reach with the Ketogenic diet.

For sure there will be many trainers and „Diet-Gurus" telling you that you have to get at least 100g of carbs everyday to prevent our brains from braking down muscles to get higher amounts of carbs. This is only true if your body is high regularly high on carbs, high on insulin and blood sugar and has no ketones to give the brain its needed energy. We said in Myth #1 that our brain can switch in „keto-mode" too, which will decrease the amount of carbohydrates needed by a lot.

The ketogenic diet is bad for your heart

Since the ketogenic diet is high in fat it is assumed that it is bad for heart health. People state that the high amount of dietary fat will increase cholesterol in the blood and lead to heart disease. As we have already seen from several studies, however, triglycerides go down, HDLs go up, blood pressure decreases, and LDLs become healthier.

Most weight loss comes from water weight

It is true that you will lose water weight in the beginning of the ketogenic diet. This is because the glycogen that you store in your liver and muscles, as a backup if your blood sugar gets low, binds to water. In addition, as blood sugar levels drop, so do insulin levels. This drop in insulin allows the kidneys to remove more sodium from the body resulting in less water retention as well. The result of these two factors working together will almost immediately cause a significant amount of water weight to be lost. There is no good reason to argue that this is a bad thing. If you don't need that extra five to ten pounds of water weight, why carry it around everywhere?

Ketogenic Dieters suffer from low fiber intake caused disease

First of all, it is more then obvious that the standard western diet contains far too less fiber to maintain a healthy intestinal flora. Second, the Ketogenic diet provides just so much variation in vegetables such as spinach, broccoli, cabbage and much more which the main source of carbohydrates for Ketogenic dieters.

Don't let Myth of people who do not have the knowledge needed bring you off your path to success!

CHAPTER 5: WHAT TO EAT AND WHAT TO AVOID UNDER LOW CARB KETOGENIC DIET

There are certain precautions you have to take when switching to Ketogenic diet for weight loss, the most important one is that you must not end your regular meals abruptly, rather you should take a gradual approach. Most of us consume meals that comprises of more than 50% carbs, and when you switch to ketogenic diets abruptly, you may have to cope with some side effects such as; Dizziness, headache, fatigue and irritability. For this reason, you should aim at cutting down your carb intake by 10-20% daily, until you comfortably switch to ketogenic diets.

Increasing your water intake can help you switch effectively into ketogenic diet phase, and the reason being that high carb diets normally increase water-retention capacity, and when you switch to Ketogenic diets, you may lose more water than usual. While some side effects of abrupt switching to ketogenic diets can be mild, most of them will disappear within few hours or days.

What to consume and what to avoid when switching to Ketogenic diets

The Ketogenic diet approach is simple and straight-forward; eat real food and avoid high carbs. You should consider eating real and nutritious foods such as eggs, meat, nuts, dairy, vegetables and fruits. From your shopping list to eating habit, Ketogenic diets must pass through everything. Here is a guide to what you should consume as Ketogenic diet:

Meat

many types of meats are recommended, these include; beef, game meat, turkey, and chicken. Make sure you mix the fatty part of the meat with the lean and skin portion. If possible, try as much as possible to consume organically raised animals, and make sure the meat is properly cleaned before cooking.

Fish

These include all kinds of fishes, and shellfish. Special choices include: Salmon, Herring and Mackerel, but try as much as possible to avoid breading.

Eggs

all kinds of eggs can be consumed but more importantly, organically raised poultry eggs are recommended. Eggs consumed as Ketogenic diet can be boiled, fried or made as Omelets.

Natural fats and high fat sauces

You may consider cooking your meals with butter and cream because they make your foods taste good and can make you feel satiated the more. Hollandaise sauce is also recommended, however, you must check all the ingredients used in making the sauce or simply make one by yourself. You can also make use of coconut or olive oil in place butter and other forms of cooking oils.

Vegetables cultivated above the ground

Vegetables that grow above the ground are excellent sources of essential minerals and vitamins. You should consider vegetables such as;

Cauliflower, Cabbage, Brussels sprouts, Broccoli, Eggplant, Asparagus, Olives, Zucchini, mushrooms, spinach, Lettuce, Avocado, Cucumber, Peppers, Onions, and Tomatoes.

Dairy foods

Dairy products must be selected if you are not allergic to some foods such as milk. If you have lactose intolerance, then you should consider talking to your doctor about alternative choices you can make. For dairy products you must select full-fat or medium-fat options such as cream (about 40% fat), butter, Greek Yoghurt, Turkish yoghurt, High-fat cheese, sour cream, and Greek cheese. You need to be careful with the use of skimmed and regular milk because they contain milk sugar. Similarly, try as much as possible to avoid flavored, low fat products, and sugary foods.

Nuts and seeds

These are highly nutritious foods with lots of protein. They can be your best companions when watching the TV, thus they are good replacements for candies and other unhealthy sugary snacks. Some of the best nuts and seeds you should consider include: peanuts and groundnuts.

Berries

Berries are okay but must be consumed in moderation, most especially if you are sensitive to them. Berries are great and delicious when consumed with whipped cream. There are no limits to the choices of berries you can consider; strawberries, Cranberries, blueberries and blackberries are some of the best.

liquids

Water is highly recommended; it keeps you hydrated even though your body's water retention capacity may be lowered while consuming Ketogenic diet. Water will sustain your system by transporting nutrients to all parts of your body. Try as much as possible to avoid caffeinated drinks because they are diuretic in nature and you may have to urinate all the time — this means you will remain dehydrated.

Try as much as possible to read the labels of all food items before buying them at the grocery stores. The rule of thumb here is that your diet should be 5% or less carbs.

What to avoid in Ketogenic dieting?

Ketogenic diet works best to help you lose weight if you stick with recommended food categories as highlighted above. You must try as much as possible to avoid or extremely limit the following:

Sugar

This is the worst of them all. Sugars come in different forms, therefore you must avoid foods and beverages such as: carbonated soft drinks, buns, cakes, pastries, sugary breakfast cereals, and ice cream. If possible, try as much as possible to avoid artificial sweeteners.

Starch

Just like processed sugars, starches also contain high carbs and must be avoided if possible. Starchy foods to avoid include: Pasta, Potatoes, Bread, rice, porridge, French fries, Potato chips, and muesli. Be careful with legumes and lentils because they contain significant amount of starch, likewise whole grain foods may contain hidden sugar. If you must consume root vegetables, then you should exercise moderation.

Margarine

Margarines are processed with some synthetic materials, including hydrogen, thus they contain a high amount of Omega-6 fatty acids – these have no health benefits in addition to the fact that they taste so bad. Margarine has been clinically linked to several diseases, including worsening of asthma symptoms, inflammatory diseases and the worsening of several other food allergies.

Fruits

If you must consume fruits, they must be half un-ripened ones, and the reason being that ripe fruits are very sweet and contains lots of sugar. You should treat ripe fruits as natural forms of candies; therefore, they must be consumed sparingly.

Once in a while, you may consider eating dark chocolate because they are made up of 70% cocoa. You must drink water or tea without sugar, and if you must take coffee, then try the one with full fat cream.

If you have sufficient amount of time to workout, especially early in the morning, then you should go for low-impact exercises. Some cardio workouts, weight-lifting or stretching exercises can keep you going and speed up your metabolism for the rest of the day.

CHAPTER 6: BENEFITS OF THE KETOGENIC DIET

Contrary to the beliefs in some quarters that Low Carb Ketogenic diet will cause high fat deposits in the body, due to the presence of low carbs and high protein and fat contents, the reverse is completely the case. The "Low carb" rule here does not mean you have to consume excess saturated fats that cause high cholesterol, it simply allows you to lower your carb supplies enough, and increase other components marginally. The main benefit of Ketogenic diet is that it forces the body to rely on stored fat and fat from diet, as the primary source of energy.

Ketogenic diet helps build more lean muscles while losing fat.

The main reason for this is that individuals placed on Ketogenic diets have been found to force their bodies to use up more water, and secondly, the lowered Insulin hormones will force the kidneys to remove excess Sodium and the combined effect of these is that there is a speedy loss of weight within the shortest possible period of time.

Ketogenic diets increase the amount of HDL cholesterols while reducing LDL cholesterol levels.

Choosing the right type of unsaturated fats in your Ketogenic diet will help increase good cholesterols (HDL cholesterols), and these are healthy for the heart and general wellbeing. Ketogenic diets also help regulate blood sugar levels while reducing the risks of insulin intolerance. When carbs are broken down, they release sugar into the blood quickly and this increases blood sugar rapidly, a condition that triggers more supply of Insulin hormones, but when Ketogenic diets replace high carb diets, less sugar are released slowly into the body, a situation that can stabilize the secretion of Insulin hormones.

Control of Blood Sugar

Keeping blood sugar at a low level is critical to manage and prevent diabetes. The keto diet has been proven to be extremely effective in preventing diabetes.

Many people suffering from diabetes are also overweight. That makes an easy weight-loss regime a natural. But the keto diet does more. Carbohydrates get converted to sugar, which for diabetics can result in a sugar spike. A diet low in carbohydrates prevents these spikes and allows more control over blood sugar levels.

Increased Energy

It's not unusual, and has become almost normal, to feel tired and drained at the end of the day as a result of a poor, carbohydrate laden diet. Fat is a more efficient source of energy, leaving you feeling more vitalized than you would on a "sugar" rush.

Weight Loss

Weight loss is the biggest reason that people begin any sort of diet in the first place, and high fat and low carb diets have been used for centuries for those who tend to carry a little extra weight. One of the greatest benefits of the ketogenic diet is that it suppresses your appetite. When you have a decreased appetite and lower insulin levels, your body's fat levels will also decrease. When you enter ketosis, you will also burn fat and use your fat storages as energy. It is a win-win for most people. On a regular diet, your body uses carbohydrates to create energy, and in return, your body stores the fat in unwanted places. On the ketogenic diet, this will not be an issue at all and you will begin to lose weight.

Increase Lifespan

Some researchers found that some patients were able to lower the oxidative stress in their body when they were on the ketogenic diet. In return, this helped increase their lifespan by increasing their health. By lowering the insulin levels and using ketones as fuel, the oxidative stress was able to decrease.

Increased Brain Function

Increased brain function is another common reason that people choose to adopt the ketogenic diet. It is thought that this diet can help improve learning skills, memory recall, clarity of thought, and other cognitive functions. In studies done on humans, it was found that the ketogenic diet was beneficial to a person's brain function even over a short period.

Mitochondrial Function

Many of our everyday functions such as immunity to common illnesses, sports performance, energy, and health are dependent on how the mitochondria in our body function. Mitochondria are the energy factories in our cells, so without them, we would not be able to function properly. Studies have found that these cells function much better while subjects are on a ketogenic diet. This is because the body is able to increase its energy levels in a more efficient, stable, and steady way while in ketosis. This is because mitochondria are specifically designed to use this fat for energy. When fat is used as the body's main source of energy, it's able to decrease any toxins, which increases energy output.

Energy

On a carb-loaded diet, you may experience what is known as a carb crash. This is because our bodies are not designed to run off excess amounts of sugars for long periods of time, hence why you often feel good after eating but are unable to sustain these energy levels through the day. When you switch to the ketogenic diet, you will experience higher, more stable energy levels throughout the day. On the ketogenic diet, you can finally say goodbye to afternoon slumps and caffeine cravings. When you switch your diet, you will have readily available fat as fuel, so you will be able to go hours without food and still maintain steady energy levels. If you are a person who is addicted to sugar and caffeine, the ketogenic diet may be the answer for you.

Digestive Health Booster

While on the ketogenic diet, you will increase the level of fiber in your diet via (mostly) non-starchy vegetables and healthy fruits. By increasing the amount of fiber in your diet, you can improve your digestive health. In addition, you will also be able to lower your risk of gastric ulcers, colorectal cancer, cramping, bloating, diarrhea, and constipation.

Endurance Performance

Studies have found that the ketogenic diet is beneficial in helping athletes increase their overall performance. This can be due to the lower lactate load in the body, as well as lowered oxidative stress when the body is fueled by fat. Other studies have found that higher levels of ketones in the blood leads to increased energy over a thirty-minute period.

Overall Health Benefits

As with any diet, the ketogenic diet can offer general health benefits within your everyday life. It can help to improve your cholesterol levels, reduce your fat and weight, and decrease your triglyceride levels. Overall, the diet offers a lot of health benefits.

As you can see, there are many incredible benefits to the ketogenic diet which can help you to change your life. Of course, as with any diet, there are certain downfalls that may be holding you back from starting the diet in the first place.

Before you begin the ketogenic diet, it's important that you go over the diet with a medical professional such as your family doctor. The ketogenic diet can be a big change that may be too much for everyone. So, while there are many benefits to this diet, it's important to follow the ketogenic diet in a way that is healthy.

Improved mental focus

The keto diet is based on protein, fats, and low carbohydrates. As we've discussed, this forces fat to become the primary source of energy. This is not the normal western diet, which can be quite deficient in nutrients, particularly fatty acids, which are needed for proper brain function.

When people suffer from cognitive diseases, such as Alzheimer's, the brain isn't using enough glucose, thus becomes lacking in energy, and the brain has difficulty functioning at a high level. The keto diet provides an additional energy source for the brain.

Because this diet does not spike blood sugar levels, the brain is kept in a stable condition. Moreover, the brain simply loves ketones as its primary source of fuel.

Reduced cravings and hunger pains

Fats are known to be filling, so this particular diet does not only curb your cravings but also reduces hunger pains.

Clearer skin

Didn't you know that the ketogenic diet can help improve the quality of your skin? Several studies suggest that people who follow the ketogenic diet often experience clearing of their acne and other skin anomalies. The ketogenic diet, aside from pushing ketosis, also drives the immune system into a frenzy thus it can help eliminate inflammation on the skin.

Before you can experience the many benefits of the ketogenic diet, it is important that you eat mostly fat. But how much fat is too much?

In order to succeed with the ketogenic diet, you don't need to eat a lot of fat. Rather, you need to smartly break down what you eat to 70-80% fat, 20-25% protein, and 5-10% carbohydrates.

You have to remember that the ratio varies depending on different people thus using an online calculator can greatly help! Make sure that you stick by your macros. The problem with most people is that they tend to eat more protein thinking that protein is always equivalent to fat. Well, not quite. Once you consume protein, the protein will be broken down into a process known as gluconeogenesis and it converts protein into carbs. So, you are back to square one.

To ensure that your body is constantly in the state of ketosis, you need to test the ketone levels in your body to know whether your body is still driving under this state or if you reverted back to your usual glucose-feeding metabolism.

There are several ways to test your body for the presence of ketones. Remember that when your body starts to burn off fats as its main energy source, ketones are spilled over into your blood and urine. And it is even present in you breathe! Since ketones are spilled all over the body, you can test either your urine or breath for its presence. You don't need to punch a tiny hole on your skin for blood testing.

CHAPTER 7: ADVERSE EFFECTS OF THE KETOGENIC DIET

Although there are many incredible benefits that come with the ketogenic diet, there are some common side effects that you need to watch out for. Any diet will come with its fair share of common issues, and most of the time, they will stem from the same underlying issues. When you begin the ketogenic diet, you will want to remember that your body is used to running a certain way.

When you begin the ketogenic diet, it is possible that a variety of symptoms may occur. Studies have shown that these symptoms stem for three underlying causes including hypoglycemia, electrolyte and mineral deficiencies, and hypothalamic-pituitary-adrenal axis dysfunction. Please, do not be put off by these big terms because they will be broken down so that you have a full understanding of what is happening to your body and how you can prevent any side effects.

Hypoglycemia

One of the underlying causes of keto-adaption is due to hypoglycemia. This issue first occurs because your body is learning how to burn fat as fuel for what may be the first time. During this phase, you will most likely feel depressed, hungry, tired, irritable, dizzy, and have brain fog. It is important to realize that these side effects are common. The good news is that they go away after the first few weeks on the diet. Below, you will find a list of common side effects caused by hypoglycemia.

Side Effects of Hypoglycemia

Keto Flu: The keto flu is one of the most common side effects, and it is exactly what it sounds like. The keto flu carries many flu-like symptoms and usually happens right when you start the diet.

Sugar Cravings: A common side effect of the ketogenic diet is that people experience intense food cravings that are high in sugar. The reason the cravings may happen is because your brain enters a sort of panic mode when you first switch your diet. During this panic mode, your brain feels that you need energy from sugar or you will die. These will subside once your body begins to produce ketones as energy. As soon as this energy switch happens, your brain and body will get over thinking you're close to death.

Drowsiness and Dizziness: Before your body becomes fully adapted to the keto diet, you may experience drowsiness or dizziness. Luckily, this is a pretty short-term effect of the keto-adaption process and you will most likely feel this way because of a lack of energy. This is especially true if your blood pressure is deregulated on your new diet. There are simple ways to fix this issue as we will be going over shortly.

Reduced Physical Performance and Strength: As you begin the ketogenic diet, your body is learning how to use a new fuel source: fat. At this point, your muscles and brain are using mitochondria as its energy production. As you switch over your diet, your body will need to learn how to use ketones. During this switch, you may experience a drop in your physical ability and strength. This is a very short-term effect but can be difficult for athletic people to endure for even a short period of time.

Strategies for Overcoming Hypoglycemia

Eat: When starting your new diet, eating properly is going to be important. It is essential to eat every three to four hours. By doing this, you will keep the hunger pangs down and your blood sugar balanced.

Drink: Along with drinking lots of water, try to drink beverages rich in minerals. This is extremely important, especially in-between meals. We suggest electrolyte drinks or even broths.

Magnesium Supplements: You may want to consider taking a magnesium supplement if you experience any side effects. By taking a supplement such as L-threonate three times a day, you may be able to reduce or lesson some of the symptoms you are experiencing.

Mineral Rich Foods: While on the ketogenic diet, you will want to use salt generously. It's also important to consume foods that are rich in minerals and that are also hydrating such as cucumbers or celery. Later on, you will learn about some of the foods that will keep you healthy on the ketogenic diet.

HPA Axis Dysfunction

Your HPA Axis consists of three different glands including your Adrenals, Pituitary Gland, and the Hypothalamus. Together, these glands are in charge of regulating the stress response in your body. As mentioned previously, the ketogenic diet will essentially put your body into panic mode because it will think you are starving, and thus dying. In response, the adrenals will begin to release cortisol which acts as a signal to release any glucose you have stored in your body to provide you with energy.

When this happens, the stores of glycogen are burned quickly, and the cycle continues.

So, what happens when this energy source is taken away? Below, you will find some of the issues caused from HPA Axis Dysfunction.

Side Effects of HPA Axis Dysfunction

Sleep Issues

One of the most common side effects caused by HPA Axis Dysfunction is sleep disruption. Due to the cortisol levels in your body, these levels will begin to fluctuate and could potentially interfere with the release of melatonin in your body. The result of this happening in your system is poor sleep quality and insomnia. The main issue is that this cortisol response is extremely helpful in emergency situations, even if your body isn't aware that there is food readily available in the fridge or at the restaurant down the road. When you are aware of what is causing your issues, it will be easier to combat insomnia.

Heart Palpitations

This can mostly be attributed to the HPA axis dysfunction and the mineral imbalances in your body. If you are experiencing heart palpitations, this is due to the abnormally high levels of cortisol in your body. When these levels are too high for too long, your body starts to build a resistance to cortisol. So, to compensate for this, your body will start to secrete more adrenaline and as the adrenaline spikes in your body, an irregular heart rhythm is created.

Strategies for Supporting your HPA Axis

Magnesium Supplements: A magnesium supplement will help to support your HPA axis, which is the root of all the issues covered here. A magnesium supplement, has been proven to cross the blood-brain barrier which will help with both your pituitary glands and your hypothalamus.

Balance Blood Sugar: Taking a magnesium supplement will also help with your hypoglycemia. By balancing your blood sugar levels, you may be able to prevent the side effects of the HPA Axis dysfunction.

Adaptogenic Herbs: If you have tried the two strategies mentioned above to no avail, consider using some adaptogenic herbs. Studies have shown that these herbs can help you to build resilience to stress. When you are able to regulate your cortisol levels, you can avoid the side effects from the dysfunction of the HPA Axis.

Mineral and Electrolyte Deficiency

Minerals and electrolytes play a vital role in regulating your body's hydration which is very important for proper nerve conductivity. When you first enter keto-adaption, most of these minerals will be excreted through your urine thanks to your HPA axis dysregulation. As you can tell, all of these side effects are intertwined. In addition to the cortisol levels in your body, the HPA axis is also in charge of regulating the excretion and retention of the minerals in your body. When the HPA axis is deregulated, it is easy to become dehydrated. Unfortunately, there are a number of side effects that manifest from this imbalance.

Side Effects of Mineral and Electrolyte Deficiency Urination

One of the most obvious signs that you have a mineral and electrolyte deficiency is more frequent urination. When you begin a low-carb diet such as the ketogenic diet, your insulin levels will begin to drop. Once this happens, you will begin to secrete more sodium through your urine. This is a normal side effect of the ketogenic diet and actually is a positive sign that you are in keto-adaption.

Constipation

If you are suffering from constipation, this is most likely because you are not maintaining a proper balance of electrolytes or minerals. The ability to pass stool is influenced by water content in your body. As you make drastic changes to your diet, the microbiome will also change your stools. This is something you will want to pay special attention to when you switch over to the ketogenic diet.

Diarrhea

Conversely, some people also report experiencing diarrhea when they first start the ketogenic diet. Although constipation is more common, this may happen due to the changing microbiome in your body. If you begin to experience diarrhea on a daily basis, try activated charcoal as a binding agent to help.

Muscle Cramping: With poor hydration and mineral imbalance, you may begin to experience muscle cramps. Muscle cramps occur when you have an imbalance in proper nerve impulse conductivity. So, if you experience frequent muscle cramps, this may be because of a mineral imbalance within your body.

Strategies for Maintaining Proper Mineral Balances and Hydration

Stay Hydrated: Many of these side effects stem from being dehydrated. When you are on the ketogenic diet, be sure to stay hydrated throughout the day by drinking a lot of water, drinks with electrolytes, and even mineral-rich broths to help release toxins from your body.

Mineral Rich Foods: If you experience side effects such as muscle cramps and constipation, remember how important your diet is. Ensure that you are consuming mineral-rich foods such as seaweed, cucumbers, leafy greens, and celery as these are all ketogenic friendly foods and great for your health.

Salt Quality: While on the ketogenic diet, the quality of salt in your diet is going to be very important. So, it's recommended that you use a high-quality salt, as this will add in the sodium and trace minerals you need in your diet. We recommend using Celtic Sea Salt or Pink Himalayan Sea Salt because they are both high in trace minerals.

Ketoacidosis

Ketoacidosis is one of the more serious complications of the ketogenic diet and is something that should be taken very seriously. Ketoacidosis refers to diabetic ketoacidosis, or DKA., and is caused by a complication of Type-one diabetes mellitus. This is a life-threatening condition that occurs when you have high levels of blood sugar and ketones. When this happens, the blood in your body becomes too acidic to function properly. For some people, this issue can occur in as little as twenty-four hours, particularly those who already have Type-one diabetes. Ketoacidosis symptoms to watch out for include:

- Confusion

- Shortness of Breath

- Fruity Breath Scent

- Tiredness

- Stomach Pain

- Vomiting

- Nausea

- Dehydration

- Frequent Urination

- Extreme Thirst

Causes of Ketoacidosis

One of the main causes of ketoacidosis is poor diabetes management. For example, you could suffer from DKA even if you miss even one insulin dose or if you get an infection or illness. Additionally, certain drugs can prevent your body from using insulin the way it is meant to be. Other factors include alcohol, stress, heart attack(s), or malnutrition.

Diagnosis Ketoacidosis

Urine Ketone Levels: >5mmol/L

Blood Ketone Levels: 1.5-3.0 + 3 mmol/L

Treatment for Ketoacidosis

If you feel that you are at risk for Ketoacidosis, seek emergency help immediately. Generally, treatment will involve screening for an infection which can be taken through fluids via mouth or vein. As a result, your doctor will most likely suggest a replacement of electrolytes, and perhaps even intravenous insulin until you can balance your blood sugar level. Regardless, you will need to seek professional help, and above all, please do not take it upon yourself to treat ketoacidosis.

Challenges in Your Lifestyle

Most of us are involved in a hectic modern lifestyle. Unfortunately, this lifestyle can lend itself to two major problems that often lead to overeating: stress and sleep deprivation. Though they're related, we'll deal with them one at a time.

Stress

Particularly if it's chronic—can not only sabotage your efforts to lose weight, but can also lead you to gain weight.

When you're stressed, it can provoke your body to enter into the fear response state (also called the flight-or-fight response), which is a natural process the body goes into when you're in a dangerous situation that requires immediate action, like facing a bear. In this situation, you need an immediate source of energy to either flee the bear or fight it.

So, your body releases adrenaline into the blood stream and increases the flow of oxygen and glucose to the brain, while also suppressing non-emergency functions like digestion. Once the danger passes, your bodily responses return to normal.

But in today's society, stress is the most common trigger of the fear response state, and stress isn't something you can fight or run away from. All too often, stress (unlike the bear) doesn't go away. Stress can become chronic, leaving you in a permanent or semi-permanent state of low-grade fear. So your body pumps out adrenaline throughout the day and suppresses your digestive functions, while also overworking your heart.

Under stress, the body—thinking it's in survival mode—releases the hormone cortisol, which makes you feel hungry. The body does this because it assumes you're going to be burning calories in order to fight or flee from the bear, and therefore burn a lot of calories that will need to be replaced. So your body starts to crave carbohydrates, because carbs provide you with energy-producing glucose. In short, your body has been tricked into thinking you need to eat, so you eat.

And gain weight.

There are numerous relaxation techniques for dealing with stress (deep breathing exercises, meditation, relaxing exercises, massage, etc.) that might help you, but they're beyond the scope of this book.

Sleep Deprivation

The busy lifestyle that produces stress can also cause sleep deprivation. In fact, stress itself can cause sleep deprivation. A lot of people suffer from stress and/or sleep deprivation without even knowing it. They might just think they're tired just from work, when in fact they aren't getting enough deep, restful sleep. They might even reach a point where they're so used to being sleep-deprived that it begins to feel normal to them.

Lack of sleep decreases the body's production of leptin, a hormone that makes you feel sated, while also triggering the production of ghrelin, a hormone that makes you feel hungry. This double whammy makes you feel hungry, even if you've eaten recently.

There are numerous causes of sleep deprivation. Among them are things that prevent you from winding down before bedtime, like watching the news—which is full of violence—or watching action or horror movies. There are numerous techniques for treating sleep deprivation, though the most common—sleeping pills—is a dangerous treatment that is only meant to be used sporadically.

But the treatments for sleep deprivation are beyond the scope of this book. There are plenty of websites devoted to dealing with stress and sleep deprivation.

Maintaining Your Good Work

Starting a weight program is largely about keeping a positive mindset and not letting setbacks discourage you. Sure, determination factors into the equation, but for some people, the real time for determination is after you've successfully started losing weight.

Yes, you heard that right. Sometimes, maintaining your good work can be harder than getting your initial success.

As they say, nothing fails like success.

If you're patting your back because you've lost ten or fifty pounds and you're starting to look good, there's a danger that you're going to relax and start sloughing off. And once you start on that path, you're in trouble.

So here are some tips for maintaining the proper attitude:

Put before-and-after photos of yourself somewhere as a reminder both of what you've accomplished and where you don't want to return.

Reward yourself regularly for your hard work, but not by eating a chocolate bar. Treat yourself to something not related to food or drink.

Yes, you can occasionally cheat slightly on your diet, but not by eating carbs, because that will confuse your body and possibly throw you out of ketosis. You could maybe give yourself a couple days a month where you cheat slightly, maybe when someone takes you out to dinner or something.

If that doesn't work, and your determination starts wavering, maybe it's time to get away for a while, or maybe you'll need to make some other change in your routine.

Remind yourself that you feel healthier now and you feel better about yourself after getting to this point.

Some people develop their own mantra that they repeat to themselves whenever they start to stray. This can re-wire your brain to stay on the straight-and-narrow.

Starting an exercise program can help, especially if it's with friends or at a gym. The gym has the advantage of prodding yourself to look good in front of new people you meet.

The gym can also be a good place to meet people who've made healthy choices and can help advise you when you start to waver. It's important to have someone to talk to who's already been through what you're going through.

Think of other ways to distract yourself from temptations that you might run into. Maybe something easy like having sugarless gum or something in your pocket, or maybe you can play a certain song when temptation starts knocking. Get creative.

CHAPTER 8: OPTIMIZING EXERCISE ON THE KETOGENIC DIET.

It quickly becomes glaringly obvious that the ketogenic diet has some absolutely enormous positives associated, with no real negatives (especially once we have adapted to the diet completely).

We have also discussed how the ketogenic can improve our physical performance and our body composition in a big way – but we haven't touched on is how we should exercise if we want to achieve a specific goal.

I am aware that many of you are not only health conscious from a dietary perspective, but also from an exercise perspective. As such, I want to briefly touch on the best ways to exercise while following the ketogenic diet if you have a specific goal in mind.

Exercising for fat loss on the ketogenic diet

We have already spent some time discussing how they ketogenic is unquestionably the optimal way of eating when fat loss is our primary goal, but it is important to realize that exercising while on the ketogenic diet can further facilitate this – resulting in more rapid and far more efficient fat loss.

While following the ketogenic diet, the body basically becomes a fat burning machine – in which it breakdown fat for energy both efficiently and effectively.

Which is why the addition of lower intensity cardiovascular exercise will be a fantastic option if we want to further enhance our current rate of fat loss.

This essentially means undertaking some form of cardiovascular exercise (it doesn't matter if it is rowing, cycling, swimming, or running) at a moderate intensity, 2-3 times per week, for 30-60 minutes per session. By moderate, I mean that it should be performed at a pace that gets your heart rate up between 60 and 80 percent of your heart rate max.

In doing so, we increase the amount of energy we are burning by a massive amount – and considering that this energy is coming entirely from fats, it will lead to a significantly larger amount of fat loss, in a shorter amount of time than if we were to use diet alone.

Exercising for muscle growth and muscle strength

Now, although we have briefly discussed the capacity to build muscle on the ketogenic diet, we haven't actually discussed the best type of exercise to facilitate this.

So taking this into consideration, there is two styles of resistance training that will get us the best results if our main priority is muscle growth – and these are training for muscle strength, and muscle hypertrophy.

Muscular strength training revolves around lifting heavy loads for lower repetitions (1-6 reps), and has a host of benefits if our goal is to increase the size of our muscle tissue.

Firstly, training for muscular strength requires heavy input from the nervous system to recruit the maximal amount of muscle fibers possible. In doing so, we can get maximal muscular contractions, which tells the body that we need this muscle tissue around.

Secondly, working with these heavier loads places the muscle tissue under huge amounts of mechanical stress. The body then needs to adapt (by increasing the size and number of its muscle fibers) to become more competent at lifting these heavy loads. This results in a subsequent increase in muscle size.

Once we have performed our muscular strength based exercises, it is time to shift towards our muscular hypertrophy based training.

Muscular hypertrophy training revolves around lifting moderately heavy weights for moderate repetitions (8-12 reps).

Performing this type of training is the perfect supplement to heavier strength based training as it places a high degree of metabolic stress on the muscle tissue, which stimulates an increased rate of muscle growth.

With this goal in mind, I should remind everyone that on training days we need to be eating in a slight caloric surplus and consuming an abundance of protein – this will make it much easier to build new muscle tissue while following the ketogenic diet.

Working out and exercising on a keto diet is absolutely possible and encouraged, but it's important that you know and understand how the body will process the energy you need. When you are first adjusting to your keto diet, the lack of carbs can make you seem groggy or tired. You might wonder how you will find the energy to exercise! The good news is that, like we've been saying all along, your body adjusts to the natural process of using ketones for energy instead of harnessing carbohydrates. It will use other energy sources, such as the high amount of high-quality fats you will be eating. When your body adjusts to the state of ketosis, you will find that your energy levels are changing and you feel much more normal and are able to exercise.

A keto diet is designed to help you lose fat. A healthy diet coupled with exercise will accelerate your weight loss. You will see your weight loss occur faster and more significantly if you are working out while following your keto diet. It's not necessary and you will still lose weight, but it will speed up the process if you have a goal in mind.

There are some people who say that your work out performance will suffer due to a keto diet because you are lacking carbohydrates. Research proves otherwise! There may be a brief amount of time while your body is adjusting to the keto diet and entering ketosis that you feel your workout is slow or sluggish.

Numerous studies have shown the equivalent performance levels for athletes before and after they started a keto diet. In fact, they were able to lose weight and keep their muscle mass relatively the same. This is most people's goal when they are on keto.

Types of Exercise on a Keto Diet

There are many types of exercise you can do when on a keto diet. When beginning your diet, your body may need a week to adapt and enter the state of ketosis. You might feel sluggish or weak until your body becomes adjusted. During the beginning stage, low-intensity workouts are best for you to perform.

Yoga

Yoga is a wonderful workout to ease your body into physical activity and even has benefits of clearing your mind and easing stress.

Stair Master: This low-intensity workout is a great way to exercise without stressing your body. It tones your hamstrings and calves.

Cycling

Low-intensity cycling is an activity that can be done with minimum energy.

Walking

Simply taking a short walk around the neighborhood can be a great way to exercise without taxing your body as you get adjusted to the keto diet.

As your body adjusts to ketosis and you feel your energy level has returned to normal, you can perform other aerobic workouts that expend more energy. Be patient with yourself because your body is adjusting to extracting energy from a new pathway and using fat for its fuel source. High intensity workouts should be scaled back until you feel your energy level can meet up with the demands of your exercise. Low to moderate intensity cardio workouts are great and encouraged to help you lose weight!

Cross Fit

This is a high intensity workout that burns sugars rather than•

fats when you need fuel during a workout. Because of this, Cross Fit users might be better off doing keto during offseason as a way to lose excess body fat so their Cross

Fit performance does not suffer.

Rowing

The rowing machine is a great way to give your body a total•

workout and tone your biceps. It combines a cardio workout with a toning benefit for your lats and arm muscles.

Heavy Weight Lifting/Power Lifting

Weightlifting, in particular, is a•

great exercise to combine with your keto diet and give your body some tone and muscle definition. A study found that in a group of men who followed a weight lifting program, the ones on a keto diet showed more of a muscle mass increase after the final week of the testing period.

Swimming

Swimming is a high intensity aerobic exercise that involves your entire body. You want to ensure you feel energetic enough to engage in this activity once your body is used to your new ketosis state.

High Intensity Training

High intensity training can be rigorous especially if you are not frequently taking breaks. Be sure you are feeling rested and energetic enough to continue training, and that you are counting your macros to have a full fat intake for energy.

You may want to avoid high intensity sports like rugby, lacrosse, soccer, or tennis that do not have enough breaks. This is because these sports are high aerobic sports that place a demand on the body for more glycogen molecules. These athletes might benefit if they have a higher carbohydrate intake to produce glucose for energy.

Some Tips to Get You Motivated!

Give your body time to adjust.

Like we've described in the book thoroughly, the keto diet is naturally going to be a change from your normal lifestyle where carbohydrates make up nearly half our daily intake. Going on the keto diet will take some adjustment and it's okay to admit that you feel slow or weak for a few days. Skip a few workouts and stay safe. Be patient with your body and realize that it will take at least 2-8 days for ketosis to occur. You don't want to force yourself into your normal workout or do something strenuous. That slow, lazy feeling will pass in a few days and you will notice your energy is back.

Do not try any new workouts when you're starting a keto diet.

This is not the time for you to try a new workout or suddenly increase the amount of weights you're lifting. The initial period of keto is sometimes called the "keto flu" because you feel sluggish and your stomach feels upset like you're battling a cold or flu. It will pass within some time as your body adjusts to burning ketones and being in a state of ketosis. Don't use this time to schedule an intense new workout or sign up for a new weight training class. Stick to what you are used to so your body is familiar with the workouts you will be doing.

Make sure you're eating enough fat.

When you're starting keto, be sure you are counting your macros and eating enough fat. It can be tough to change our previous assumptions of seeing too much fat as bad for your body, but with keto, that assumption changes! If you're not eating enough high-quality fat content, it can actually harm your body and cause you to lose muscle mass. You need to compensate for the low carbohydrates intake with a high fat intake so you can urge your body into a state of ketosis. Make sure your fats are high quality and healthy fat sources like grass-fed meats, coconut or avocado oil, fish, and full fat butter and cheeses.

Skip high intensity workouts until you are fully adjusted to keto.

As we mentioned above, high intensity exercises use glycogen molecules as fuel no matter how you have your macro intake divided. Glycogen is fueled by the intake of carbohydrates. And with keto, you're in taking a low amount of carbs. Because of this, your high intensity workouts could potentially suffer, though this depends on person to person. We recommend staying away from high intensity workouts until you feel your body and energy level have fully acclimated to a keto lifestyle. Instead, we encourage moderate intensity exercise because that is the best combination to help you burn off fat. Weight lifting and cardio exercises are also great complements to a keto diet.

Don't under eat!

If you aren't following keto correctly, then you are putting your body in detrimental damage. You should not be cutting off calories that your body needs to exercise. The keto diet is full of healthy fats so you can suppress your appetite. That's why counting macros is so important to ensure you are not shortchanging yourself. If you're incorrectly reducing your calories then working out, you will feel like you do not have the energy and not getting your desired results.

Don't slam your body with unnecessary calories.

Some people think that after working out, you should consume protein shakes in that small window of time. But science shows that it takes almost 4-8 hours after we work out for muscle growth to occur. That's when the body begins to synthesize the protein that we eat to enlarge muscles after a workout. It's all about eating well and ensuring you have enough protein throughout the day to ensure your workouts are successful.

Spread out your workouts.

Doing too much during one day is taxing when it comes to anything, but especially when working out. Spread out your workouts so you are doing weight lifting 2-3 times a week, and then cardio exercises 2-3 times a week, but not doing them on the same days. You don't want to overexert your body or cause muscle damage or injury. And don't be scared to take a rest day! Your muscles and bodies need time to relax in order to grow.

Remind yourself of all the other positives of working out.

On a keto diet, after an initial drop in weight, your weight loss might plateau as you near your goal weight. That's because your body has all the calories it requires and is able to expend it for energy. It can feel discouraging to know you're not losing more weight despite exercising. Remind yourself of all the other health benefits a keto diet coupled with exercise can provide you. You reduce your body's resistance to insulin, lower inflammation, reduce stress levels, helps get a better night's sleep, improve your mood and memory, and lower your risk of heart disease. There are many benefits that keto provides and you are taking advantage of them!

Listen to your body and your doctor.

The first couple of weeks on keto can be a tough experience as your body adjusts to the new macro formula. If you feel tired or dizzy even after the initial period, it's important you rest and not perform extra physical activity or workouts. Eat carbs if that's what you need to feel better, and speak to your doctor about how you are feeling and what you may have been doing wrong. Your health is a priority and you should listen to your body!

CHAPTER 9: KETOGENIC DIET AND COMMON DISEASES

Keto Diet and Cancer

Cancer has turned into a serious disease in our modern society. While cancer was not a large factor before the 20th century (it did exist, of course), our modern diet and sedentary lifestyle have made cancer the second primary cause of death, with 1600 American dying from this disease every day. It appears that our bodies do not react well to being exposed to daily toxins.

Cancer is another reason people adopt the ketogenic diet and why it continues to gain popularity. Scientists believe that cancer cells are able to thrive on glucose as their main fuel resource. On the ketogenic diet, this source of glucose is taken away and deprives the cancer cells of the energy it needs to thrive. In one 2012 study, ten patients were put on a ketogenic diet and after 28 days, one patient experienced partial remission, five were able to stabilize, and four showed continued progress.

While any cancer treatment must be guided by your physician, it is a good idea to discuss the keto diet and what it can do to help in the treatment of this disease.

A cancer-specific keto diet may consist of as much as 90 percent fat. There is a very good reason for that. What doctors do know is that cancer cells feed off carbohydrates and sugar. This is what helps them grow and multiply in number.

As we have seen, the keto diet dramatically reduces our carbohydrate and sugar consumption as our metabolism is altered. What the keto diet does, in essence, is remove the "food" on which cancer cells feed and starves them. The result is that cancer cells may die, multiply at a slower rate, or decrease.

Another reason why a keto diet is able to slow down the growth of cancer cells is that by reducing calories, cancer cells have less energy to develop and grow in the first place. Insulin also helps cells grow. Since the keto diet lowers insulin level, it slows down the growth of tumorous cells.

When on the keto diet, the body produces ketones. While the body is fueled by ketones, cancerous cells are not. Therefore, a state of ketosis may help reduce the size and growth of cancer cells.

The keto diet may help prevent cancer from occurring in diabetic patients in the first place. People with diabetes have a higher risk level to develop cancer due to elevated blood sugar levels. Since the ketogenic diet is extremely effective at decreasing the levels of blood sugar, it may prevent the initial onset of cancer.

From what research has discovered so far, ketogenic diet may:

1. Stop the growth of cancer cells.

2. Help replace cancerous cells with healthy cells.

3. Change the body's metabolism and enable the body to "starve" cancer cells by depriving them of needed nutrition.

4. By lowering the body's insulin level, the ketogenic body may prevent the onset of cancer cells.

Keto Diet and IBS (Irritable Bowel Syndrome)

If you suffer from IBS, the thought of being on a high-fat diet may seem like a bad idea, and, in fact, eating more fat will most likely end in bouts of diarrhea at first. Some studies have found that a diet which incorporates less sugar can provide relief to those who suffer from IBS and even improve stool habits, quality of life, and abdominal pain.

Keto Diet and Blood Sugar

One of the healthiest side benefit of the Keto Diet is that it regulates your blood sugar. Okay, you're thinking, that's great and all, but why is that such an important part of my overall health?

When you think 'blood sugar,' you've got to also think about your body's energy that's processed as part of your overall metabolism. Your blood moves along the interior highway of your artery and vein system, carrying nutrients from the food you eat to every part of your body.

However, just like a polluted river, blood can also become clogged with too much glucose. That glucose wasn't processed by your liver, so it ends up in your blood stream, elevating your blood sugar levels. The sugars and carbs you eat end up in your blood stream, spiking your energy levels.

You spike your blood sugar; you receive a spike of energy. That doesn't seem so bad. A quick burst of energy is good from time to time. But with every spike comes an opposite reaction of the crash. That crash is not healthy and represents too much of a change in your blood sugar. It also makes you feel sluggish, mentally foggy, drained, and it also interferes with your natural sleep cycle. As a result, in order to feel that burst of energy again, you're naturally going to – you guessed it – reach for something else to spike your blood sugar.

If you repeat this spike-crash-spike-crash cycle too often, you're sending your blood sugar on an unnecessary and unhealthy roller coaster that can have long-term negative consequences.

Keto diet and Acne

While most of the benefits of a keto diet are well-documented, one benefit catches some people by surprise: better skin and less acne. Acne is fairly common. Ninety percent of teens suffer from it, and many adults do, as well.

If you suffer from acne, the ketogenic diet may be beneficial for you. This is because studies have shown that foods high in glycemic are one of the reasons that acne outbreaks are stimulated, so when you are eating foods that are lower in glycemic on the ketogenic diet, you reduce your chances of developing acne.

While it was always thought that acne was at least exacerbated by poor diet, controlled research is still being conducted. However, many people on the keto diet have reported clearer skin. There may be a logical reason.

In addition, acne thrives on inflammation. The ketogenic diet eases and reduces inflammation, thus enabling the body to decrease acne eruptions. Fatty acids, which are found in abundance in fish, are a known anti-inflammatory.

While research is still being done, it seems likely that a keto diet has beneficial effects for clearer, healthier, more glowing skin.

Keto and Anti-Aging

Many diseases are a natural result of the aging process. While there have not been studies done on humans, studies on mice have shown brain cell improvement on a keto diet.

Several studies have shown a positive effect of the keto diet on patients with Alzheimer's disease. What we do know is that a diet filled with good nutrients and antioxidants, low in sugar, high in protein and healthy fats, while low in carbohydrates, enhances our overall health. It protects us from the toxins of a poor diet.

There is also research indicating that using fatty acids for fuel instead of sugar may slow down the aging process, possibly because of the negative effects that sugar has on our overall wellbeing.

In addition, the simple act of eating less and consuming fewer calories is a matter of basic health, as it prevents obesity and its inherent side effects.

So far, studies have been limited. However, considering the powerful positive effects of the ketogenic diet on our health, it is logical to assume this diet will help us grow older in a more natural way while delaying the natural effect of aging. A normal western diet laden with sugars and processed foods are certainly detrimental to warding off the signs of aging.

Keto and Eyesight

Diabetics are aware that high blood sugar can lead to a higher risk of developing cataracts. Since the keto diet controls sugar levels, it can help retain eyesight and help prevent cataracts. This has been proven in several studies involving diabetic patients.

Keto diet and Alzheimer's

People who have Alzheimer's suffer from a condition where their brain is unable to use glucose. As a result, this often leads to high levels of inflammation, and some scientists even refer to this as "type 3" diabetes. Thus, the ketogenic diet is incredibly beneficial if the brain is unable to use glucose. By using ketones, this may assist those who have Alzheimer's.

Keto diet and Autism

We know the keto diet affects brain functions. In a study on autism, it was found that it also has a positive effect on autism. Thirty autistic children were placed on the keto diet. All showed improved in autistic behavior, especially those on the milder autistic spectrum. While more studies are needed, the results were extremely positive.

Keto diet and GERD (Gastro esophageal Reflux Disease)

Individuals who were on the ketogenic diet, even if it was for less than week, were able to lower the acidity in their esophagus. These people reported that their heartburn conditions were less severe while on the ketogenic diet. These reductions were most likely linked to upping their fat and lowering the amount of carbohydrates in their diet.

Keto diet and Headaches and Migraines

For some, switching to the ketogenic diet also helps to decrease the number of migraines they experience. Additionally, it was found that the ketogenic diet helped to reduce the number of drugs people used to help with their headache and migraine symptoms.

Keto Diet and Epilepsy

The initial use of the keto diet had nothing to do with weight loss or diabetes management, for which it is now so well-known. Instead, the diet was created by a doctor in 1924 to help his patients suffering from epilepsy. Epilepsy is a nervous system disorder that can bring on recurrent seizures at any time. The symptoms can be spasms and convulsions, or an unusual psychological view of the world. In any case, it is caused by abnormal brain activity. The severity of the symptoms varies from person to person. A person is diagnosed with epilepsy only if he or she suffers from more than two seizures in one full day. Anyone can suffer from this disorder, but it seems to affect young children the most, perhaps because the young brain is still in a state of development.

However, people who used the keto diet to treat seizures continued seeing remarkable success. Today, doctors are returning to using the low carbohydrate, high-fat diet to treat their patients. The results have been extremely promising.

For anyone with children who experience seizures, the inclusion of a keto diet in the child's treatment should be discussed with his or her physician.

Keto Diet and Blood Pressure

The symptoms of high blood pressure can be caused by an overload of carbohydrates in the diet, more than the body is able to handle. As we've discussed, carbohydrates are converted into sugars, which raise the body's blood sugar level, forcing the body to create additional insulin. Insulin stores fat, and an excess of insulin can lead to obesity. All of this can have a negative effect on your blood pressure. While this is a major benefit for weight loss, it's also beneficial for those who suffer from high blood pressure.

Consuming fewer carbohydrates decreases both the level of insulin and the blood pressure level. This simple dietary change can make a huge difference in your blood pressure. The people were divided into two groups. One group was put on a ketogenic diet containing a maximum of 20 grams of carbohydrates, while the other group was given the weight-loss drug orlistat, in addition to being counseled to follow a low-fat regimen.

Both groups showed similar weight loss. What surprised the researchers was that half of the keto group showed a decrease in blood pressure, while only 21 percent of the low-fat diet group had any decrease in blood pressure. While weight loss itself would bring about a lowering of blood pressure, the study suggests that a decrease in carbohydrate intake can help lower blood pressure even more.

It was found that potassium specifically had a huge effect on lower hypertension. Doctors recommend at least 4,700 mg of potassium each day for anyone wishing to lower his or her blood pressure.

CHAPTER 10: HOW TO MAKE A MENU OF KETO DIET?

Grocery list for your perfect Keto plan

Fats

Fats will be the biggest part of your daily calorie intake, so we will start with analyzing them. When you are making choices on which food to eat, always keep in mind your personal taste. The important thing is to select the right types of fats and avoid the wrong ones that disrupt your metabolism.

Here are some suggestions on what you should include in your ketogenic diet: - Duck fat - Grass-fed butter - Tallow - Ghee - Egg yolks - Macadamia - Olive - Avocado - Fish (salmon, trout, tuna, sardines) and animal fat (non-hydrogenated) - Oils: olive, coconut, macadamia, MCT (choose cold-pressed oils) Now, here is a list of fats to avoid as they are not healthy for your body: - Refined oils: canola, sunflower, soybean, corn, grape seed - Margarine – even the "heart healthy" one is not good for your health and leads to weight gain and increases stroke risk

Vegetables

Although vegetables are important for a ketogenic diet, you need to make smart choices when it comes to choosing them. The general rule for vegetables is to focus on the leafy green ones.

I will now list the types of vegetables you can freely consume. I suggest you focus on the first several items on the list and limit the intake of root vegetables and nightshades because of their carb amounts: - Dark, leafy green vegetables – spinach, lettuce, Swiss chard and kale - Vegetables that have lower carb levels – celery, cucumber, zucchini, squash, asparagus - Cruciferous vegetables – broccoli, cabbage, Brussels sprouts - Nightshades – tomatoes, eggplant, and peppers - Root vegetables – garlic, onion, radishes - Sea vegetables – Kombu and nori You might think that all types of vegetables are healthy, but some of them have high carb levels that make them a bad choice for a ketogenic diet. These are: - Peas, potatoes, corn, parsnips, yucca, yams, beans and legumes

Proteins

There is a wide variety of sources for your protein. The darker meat is a bit fattier than the white meat, but the only rule you should stick to is to be careful not to over-consume on protein. The goal of ketogenic diet is the state of ketosis, but a higher intake of protein than the one recommended might lower your body's ability to produce ketones and increase the production of glucose.

Here is the list of proteins to eat while you are on keto diet: - Meat from pasture-raised or grass-fed animals - Fish – preferably wild caught, such as catfish, halibut, cod, mackerel, salmon, tuna, trout or snapper - Shellfish – lobsters, clams, oysters, mussels, scallops, squid - Organic eggs – they contain a lot of vitamins and fatty acids The main thing to avoid is eating processed ingredients, which is why you should steer clear of: - Products from factory-farmed animals and seafood – they are lower in nutrients and more often than not contain preservatives that can cause cancer and affect your health in a negative way

Dairy Products

Dairy provides you with an easy way to add additional fats to your meals. You can be creative and combine them with other food as long as you watch out your protein intake. People who are lactose intolerant should naturally stick to those products that contain less lactose.

The examples of full-fat dairy product you should eat while on a ketogenic diet are: - Cottage cheese, goat cheese, mozzarella, cheddar and other soft and hard cheeses - Yoghurt - Sour cream - Homemade Mayonnaise Remember, it is a much healthier option to choose raw and organic dairy products.

The dairy products you should avoid include: - Milk – it is high in carbs - Low-fat products-usually overly processed and stripped of fatty acids and other nutrients

Fruits

Fruits usually have a high amount of carbs or sugar and they are not recommended during a ketogenic diet. The only exceptions are avocados and berries, such as blueberries or raspberries, but you should also limit their intake. The same goes for citrus fruit, such as oranges and lemons and their juices (and zest).

Nuts and Seeds

They a good fat source, but they also have a considerable amount of carbs and proteins, so you need to be careful with the amount you consume. You can use raw nuts to add texture or flavoring to the meals. In general, nuts and seeds should be roasted because that takes away all the anti-nutrients.

These are some nuts and seeds you can consume during keto: - Macadamia/Brazil nuts, walnuts, pecans, almonds, sunflower and flax seeds - Flour made from nut and seed is an excellent replacement for regular flour. You can try almond or coconut flour Aside from limiting the number of nuts and seeds you can consume, you should also avoid: - Cashews, chestnuts, pistachios and peanuts because of higher carb levels

Spices

This is a real tricky part as you want to add flavor to your food, but you don't want to make a mistake and significantly increase your intake of carbs.

The important thing when it comes to spices is to read the label because most of the pre-made mixes have added sugar, which is recommended to avoid.

You can safely use: - Chili powder - Cayenne pepper - Oregano - Cinnamon - Cumin - Basil - Parsley - Thyme - Rosemary - Cilantro Please note that spices contain carbs and you need to make sure to add them to your calculations.

The good news is that you can freely use salt and pepper as much as you like and there is no need to worry about their nutritional information.

Sweets

Believe it or not, most or the cravings in our organism are caused by sugar. Your cravings can get particularly strong during a ketogenic diet. If you can endure, it is a great idea to restrain from any sweeteners for 30 days. This way you will be able to completely eliminate cravings.

However, this might be a tricky job, so take a look at some sweets that are allowed even if you are on a ketogenic diet: - Dark chocolate with 70% cocoa is rich in antioxidants - Inulin – a sweet plant that helps with your blood sugar level - Stevia, xylitol and similar sweeteners, but don't go for powdered versions but the pure products Naturally, you should limit the intake of sweets. More important than anything, this is sweet food you should avoid on a keto diet: - Sugar - Honey - High-fructose corn syrup These have high amounts of sugar and can easily knock you out of ketosis.

Sauces

The best sauces and other condiments are made from scratch. Pre-made sauces often have added sugars, which aren't a healthy option for your body, especially if you are on a ketogenic diet.

You should think about using a thickener, such as a xanthan gum or guar. It provides a good way to thicken watery sauces and keep them healthy.

Aside from the pre-made sauces, you can use these condiments as long as you read the ingredients: - Ketchup (no added sugar) - Mayonnaise (homemade, if possible) - Mustard - Hot sauce - Sauerkraut - Relish - Worcestershire sauce - Horseradish - Caesar, ranch and other fattier salad dressings

Drinks

Aside from having to eat, you will also have to drink something. In fact, staying hydrated is an important part of every ketogenic diet.

Here are what drinks are allowed: - Water – your go-to source and the most important way of staying hydrated. Aside from still, you can also drink sparkling water - Coffee and tea – it improves your concentration, but do not add sugar or milk.

On the other hand, you should make sure not to consume: - Soft drinks, including diet sodas - Craft beers and sweet wines, as well as flavored liquor, keep in mind that alcohol slows down the process of losing weight - Fruit juices

How to make the menu?

Despite the fact that on the internet you can find many ready-mades compiled menus and even more books with recipes, I would like to teach you to make your own menu, because it's very simple and takes very little time. When you master the basic rules your fantasy flight in keto-kitchen will be unlimited. Making a menu is easy.

The main principle stated above is that you need to eat protein + fat and not to eat carbohydrates.

We take products of animal origin (meat, fish, poultry, eggs, cottage cheese). Dairy products with a mass fat content more than 1.5% prohibited. Just choose those products where there are no carbohydrates!

So, for example the protein content, fat and calorie content in some products (per 100 grams) is lean Pork: 15 g protein + 30 g fat = 330 CCAL

Mackerel: 18 g protein + 9 g fat = 153 CCAL Salmon: 21 g protein + 15 g fat = 219 CCAL

One Egg (with yellow): 6-8 g protein + 6 g fat = 88 CCAL

We do the same with vegetables:

Cucumbers: 1 G Protein + 0 G Fat (4 CCAL) + 3 G Carbohydrates = 16 CCAL

Calculate the total amount of consumed products so that according to grams weight protein = weight of fat.

Of course, the caloric content of fat will be twice more than in protein, but this is exactly what we need to keep the right proportion.

For example, 100 g of non-fat pork (15 g protein + 30 g fat) + 100 g mackerel (18 g protein + 9 g fat) = 33 g protein + 39 g fat, i.e. The weight of proteins is almost equal to the weight of fat, and we need it.

You can make a menu for any products in this way! In any quantity you need. Then the total amount of the resulting meal is divided into 6-7 servings. In the end, you get your daily diet. It's not difficult at all! Make it once and then using the results all time.

You can prepare delicious salads:

- boiled shrimp + arugula + boiled eggs + olive oil with a few drops of lemon juice;

- tomatoes + cucumbers + soft cheese + vegetable oil;

- Shrimp, mussels, octopus and squid boiled and fried in butter just sprinkle with apple cider vinegar.

If it is a question of hot dishes, then for a keto diet the following is suitable:

- Baked fish in foil - this can be salmon, trout, or mackerel. Add only the greens of dill, a few slices of lemon, a pinch of salt, and ground pepper.

- Roast meat with onions and fennel fruits - everything fit to the brazier / mold, filled with fat cream and stewed in the oven or on the stove for an hour. For this dish it will be appropriate to serve fresh cucumbers or arugula leaves.

You can make a casserole of cottage cheese and eggs, or prepare a magnificent omelet in the oven. In the first case, you need to mix 1 kg of cottage cheese with 5 eggs, put it in a mold and top it with fatty sour cream, bake 20 - 30 minutes on medium heat and the omelet is made even easier: you need to beat eggs and milk in equal quantities by volume, salt and pour into a mold. After 15 minutes' blend in the oven, a hot dish will be ready for lunch or dinner.

The weight of proteins and fats in each serving does not need to be equal. The main thing is that your total daily intake follows the caloric content (1/3 of proteins + 2/3 fats, remember?) You can eat only pork in one meal, and in another eat mackerel, for example. It makes sense only to have a daily calorie content!

Features of Keto Diet for Vegans

In the vegan ketogenic diet, the same principles apply as in the classical diet: a reduction in the amount of carbohydrates and an increase in fat. All fast carbohydrates, such as sugar, white cereals, and flour, are uniquely removed, a large amount of sweet fruits, dried fruits and sweeteners (including unrefined ones).

Fats should be consumed first of all in the form of avocados, seeds, and nuts, which are rich with fat and protein, and oils of cold pressing of the highest quality (olive, coconut, pumpkin, walnut).

A strict vegan ketogenic diet also excludes all cereals, legumes and sweet starchy vegetables such as sweet potato, potatoes, beets, pumpkin.

The basis of the diet is green and non-starchy vegetables, mushrooms, nuts, seeds, berries, fermented foods, algae and quality fats of all types.

Remember that nuts should be soaked, especially if you consume them in large quantities. Otherwise, the phytic acid contained in them can interfere into the process of assimilation of nutrients from other products. It will be even better if you can sprout seeds and nuts - this greatly increases the amount of micro-and macronutrients in the product, making them more bioavailable.

When you are switching to a ketogenic vegan diet, you need to change your habits, buy all the necessary products and learn new ways of cooking them.

A strict ketogenic diet implies a reduction in the amount of carbohydrates to 20 grams per day, which is almost impossible on veganism, with maintaining health. Focus on the maximum level of 50 grams of carbohydrates per day - this figure is quite realistic if you exclude cereals, legumes, and fruits.

Also (especially at the beginning) careful planning of your meals will avoid situations in which you cannot find the right foods and make yourself a balanced meal.

I recommend regularly donating blood for analysis to prevent imbalance of micro-and macro elements. If necessary, you can use them as supplements or vitamins.

Below are some dishes that you can prepare on a ketogenic vegan diet.

Breakfast:

- pudding from chia seeds or flaxseeds on nut or coconut milk with a handful of berries,

- smoothies with vegan protein, avocado, herbs, lemon juice,

- pancakes with almond flour and berries.

Dinner:

- a large green salad with whole avocado, broccoli and walnuts

- scramble of tofu with spinach and mushrooms

- zucchini "noodles" with mushrooms and nut sauce.

Snack:

- a handful of "activated" nuts

- smoothies with tea matte, coconut milk and almond

- a handful of berries (if you did not eat them for breakfast).

Dinner:

- gazpacho with hemp seeds and crackers from flax and nuts

- "pizza" from zucchini and flaxseed with avocado and a large green salad with olives

- "rice" from cauliflower with cashew cream.

Like many others, the ketogenic vegan diet should be selected individually and take into account not only the characteristics of your body but also your lifestyle, goals and taste preferences. This diet can be maintained for several weeks, and you can make it a way of life, with periods including more carbohydrates in the form of cereals. The main thing is that all those changes bring you joy, pleasure, and positively affect your health and well being.

CHAPTER 11: MISTAKES THAT CAN KEEP YOU FROM BEING SUCCESSFUL ON YOUR KETOGENIC DIET

Numerous studies have pointed out the benefits of following the ketogenic diet. While some people experience successful results, others experience weight loss plateau. This term is defined as the certain stage wherein the body stops losing weight. Honestly, I have experienced weight loss plateau in the past and it is kind of frustrating that you worked so hard, but the extra pounds are not coming off. If you have experienced or is experiencing this problem, have you ever wondered what is it that you are doing wrong? And you are actually right. There is something that you are doing wrong that is why this diet is not working for you now. Thus, below are common ketogenic diet mistakes that you need to be aware of and avoid. When talking about the keto diet, it's only natural we hit upon what are some common mistakes. They may seem like little things but they can add up when it comes to increasing your carbohydrate count or causing you to overeat and consume too many calories. Here are some of the mistakes to look out for.

Using the keto diet as a "quick fix" diet method

After hearing about the millions of successful weight loss stories of people following the keto lifestyle, some are tempted to use keto as a quick way to lose some weight and then go back to their normal lifestyle. That's not how keto is meant to work. It is a long-term lifestyle change that incorporates aspects of a healthy diet and active lifestyle to guide your body towards your goal weight. Being on keto for just a few weeks might help you shed a few pounds, but if you abandon the diet, then you will gain back the pounds. It's not meant to be a quick fix, but a lifestyle change that helps you lose weight and improve your overall health.

Not replenishing your body's Sodium levels

One of the effects of consuming a low carb Ketogenic diet is that it reduces Insulin levels and one of the main functions of Insulin is to direct cells to store fats. Another major function of insulin is to instruct the kidneys to hold firmly unto its sodium. When you consume low carb Ketogenic diets for a very long time, your insulin levels go low and your body loses more sodium alongside substantial amount of water-this is one of the reasons why most people often get rid of bloating even within the first 24 hours of consuming low carb diets.

You need to keep in mind that sodium is a key electrolyte in the body, and the excess shedding of it from the kidneys can create a serious health risk. The excess shedding of sodium may result in some slight issues such as light-headedness, headaches, fatigues and constipation, especially during the first few days of Ketogenic dieting. The only way to avoid this problem is to increase slightly, your salt intake (you may also consume broth once in a while). This will help you increase your sodium level significantly.

Consuming too much protein

You need to keep in mind that the main goal of low carb Ketogenic diet is to consume healthy fat and not protein, as we all know that protein is an important macro-nutrient that can improve satiety while increasing fat burning. With this believe, more protein should definitely lead to weight loss and improve drastically your body composition, but the problem is that low carb dieters who consume lean animal proteins will end up eating too much of it and when you eat more protein than your body needs, your body will convert the excess into Glucose and this will prevent your body from getting into "Ketosis" phase. Your body will not burn sufficient fat to cause you to lose weight until it enters the Ketosis phase, thus you need to limit your protein consumption to 15% or less of your total diet. An ideal formulated Ketogenic diet should have low carb with high fat and moderate protein

Consuming more carbs than recommended levels

Some people don't stick with the recommended <5% carb for Ketogenic diet. Some may be confused at what exactly constitute a low carb diet by estimating that anything less than 150g of carb a day is "low carb". There may be no problem if you get 150g of carbs a day from unprocessed carbohydrate foods, but quick drinks such as carbonated soft drinks and ripe fruits can sharply increase your carb intake, causing you to take more than necessary and this can lead to an increase in blood glucose, with a resultant effect of increase in Insulin levels.

Not being patient

Low carb Ketogenic diet is not a "quick" weight loss program that will make you lose fat immediately, it takes some dedication and consistencies to make it work for you. People often get into stumbling blocks when they expect too much within a short period of time. There is one thing you need to understand about Ketogenic diets, first, your body was designed to preferentially burn carbs instead of fat, especially when carbs are available. So, if you always make carbs available, that is what your body will burn. if you drastically reduce your carb intake, your body will automatically shift to another source of energy — in most cases, fats. The fat that your body breaks down must come either from your diet or from the stored fats in your body.

Full adaptation of the body to low carb Ketogenic diet may take between few days to weeks but it will eventually yield results once your body has shifted focus to burning fat. You need to be patient to reap the full benefits of low carb Ketogenic diets.

Being afraid to eat fat (eating high fat diets)

Stereotype thinkers will make you believe that eating fat is bad and we all have been told to always avoid fat since we were little, but now that the truth has been revealed through Ketogenic diets, you are now aware that the best possible way to lose weight is to switch your body into a fat-burning mode, instead of carb-burning mode. Though it is ideal to avoid bad cholesterol, including those found in vegetable oils and fast foods, these fats may increase your chances of developing inflammation and wouldn't aid your weight loss either. Try as much as possible to replace vegetable oil with coconut oil, beef bacon grease and butter.

Trying to impose too many changes at once

You need to recognize that some addictive lifestyles can be very difficult and challenging to change. For instance trying to dump a sedentary lifestyle filled with consumption of junk foods to a completely Ketogenic lifestyle of low carb should take a period of preparation because you don't want to put too much pressure on your body within a short period of time. Statistics and researches have shown that individuals who prepare enough before the commencement of ketogenic diets often end up making the biggest successes of weight loss.

Being afraid of eating high-fat content

One of the changes you have to make on the keto diet is overcoming what society has told you about eating a lot of fat. For this diet, it's that healthy fat content that helps you lose weight! When it comes to your macronutrients count, about 75% of them will be coming from fat. Don't be afraid of how much fat you are eating, but be aware of choosing healthy, grass-fed, organic fats and butter so you are eating the best quality fat to help induce your body to a state of ketosis.

Obsessing over your weight

That's easier said than done especially when one of your goals for going on the keto diet is losing weight. But checking your weight multiple times a day or obsessing over why you aren't losing weight yet is not productive and will not motivate you. Instead, focus on eating right and incorporating exercise into your day. That's how you will see a drop in the numbers on the scale and you will physically feel better. If you strength train, you might even see a slight increase because your fat is being transformed into muscle weight. It's important that you be patient and take account of your situation and your lifestyle before worrying that you aren't hitting your target weight goal yet.

Not Transitioning Slowly Enough to the Diet

Too many people want to jump right in and make big changes so they can lose a lot of weight in a hurry. This can produce a lot of stress on your body and your emotions. For one thing, it can cause bladder issues, making you go to the bathroom frequently. You should transition slowly to this diet, gradually increasing your fat intake and lowering your carb and protein intakes over the first two or three weeks until you arrive at the proper ratios. This will allow your body the time it needs to make a smooth transition to the ketosis state.

Obsessing about Your Ketone Levels

Though it's a good idea to keep track of your levels, worrying about them only makes things worse, possibly leading to depression. For the first few weeks, maintaining a positive state of mind is critical for your long-term success. On this diet, you want your body to feel good during the transition period, so the less stress and disappointment you feel, the better you'll make it through the transition. If you make it through the transition period with a positive attitude, you'll soon start burning layers of fat off.

Eating the Wrong Fats

Avoid oils made from vegetables or seeds. Use saturated fats like animal fats, coconut oil and butter. Monounsaturated fats like olive oil are also good. Nuts are another good food.

Focusing Solely on Eliminating Carbs

Though cutting back on carbs is important, completely eliminating them is probably not be a good idea. Some people need more carbs than others, and certain carbs—like non-starchy vegetables—are quite good for the body, especially those that are high in fiber. Moderation and variety in the diet can be beneficial not only to your body but for your emotional satisfaction and well-being.

Overeating Protein

It might seem like if you're eating fewer carbohydrates, why not eat more protein to fill that gap in your diet? But this is actually counterintuitive because it has negative effects on your body if you are following a keto lifestyle. Your body only needs a certain amount of protein a day. When you hit that limit, the excess protein is actually stored as fat. This is not good because that's more fat that you have to burn off! Focus on your macronutrients count and use an app tracker to count your calories throughout the day. This keeps you focused and aware of how much you are eating of each food group and you can make changes to your diet as necessary.

Though protein is absolutely essential for maintaining your organs and muscles, eating too much can hinder or even prevent your body from entering ketosis, because excess protein can be converted into glucose. So remember to monitor your protein intake closely, eating neither too little nor too much of it.

Not Eating Sufficient Amounts of Fat

It's tough for most dieters to get used to the idea of eating a lot of fat, but you need to do it for this diet to work. So just enjoy all the yummy fat without feeling guilty about it.

Overeating Processed Foods

The Keto Diet emphasizes eating natural foods. Yes, natural foods take longer to prepare, but if you plan your meals ahead of time and make sure you have the ingredients handy, it saves you quite a bit of time in running to the store. Occasionally eating a little processed is okay for a little variety, but it isn't real food.

Not Getting Sufficient Salt, Minerals and Vitamins

Sometimes, people on this diet are so concerned about getting the proper proportions of fat, protein and carbs that they forget about basic nutrients. And yes, a little salt is good for the body. Too much salt can cause inflammation in a person who eats too many unnatural foods, but eating a couple teaspoons a day on a natural diet is fine.

Consuming Too Much Alcohol

Drinking alcohol not only adds unnecessary carbs and bad sugars to your diet, but can also interfere with your body's ability to remain in ketosis. While it's okay to occasionally indulge a little, it's best to keep alcohol to a minimum.

Eating on Too Rigid of a Schedule

While a family meal schedule can sometimes be necessary in our hectic modern lives, it's important on this diet to listen to the needs of your body. Whenever possible, if you're hungry, eat. If you aren't, don't. The body is a lot wiser than we give it credit for, and trying to impose your own schedule upon it can throw off your body's rhythms.

Not Committing Yourself Fully to the Diet

Maintaining the proper proportions of fat to carbs is important. If you continually slack off and allow yourself to indulge in extra carbs, you can wind up with a high-fat, high-carb diet, which can not only terminate your ketosis and quickly add pounds, but can be harmful to your health.

Obsessing about Your Cholesterol Levels

Many people believe that cholesterol is bad, while in fact it's essential for your body. The doctor who originally came up with the idea that cholesterol leads to heart disease eventually rejected the idea after examining the research on the subject.

Believing the Keto Diet Is a Quick Fix

The diet isn't a quick fix that will cure whatever ails you and instantly start burning off a lot of fat. Forget all the commercials about miracle diets that burn x number of pounds in x number of days. Not only are those stories questionable, but many of those testimonials are from people who eventually put a lot of those pounds back on.

Not Being Prepared for the Onset of Ketosis

Some people get the "Keto flu" when they first enter ketosis. Typical symptoms are any or all of the following: headache, stomach ache, nausea, fatigue, sleepiness and lack of mental clarity. Symptoms can last from a day to a week. You can usually avoid this by transitioning to the new diet over a period of two or three weeks. Drinking lots of water helps prevent the keto flu, mainly because entering ketosis can cause you to urinate more frequently. You can also lose electrolytes like sodium, magnesium and potassium in your urine, so make sure you replace those electrolytes. Transitioning slowly to the new diet can also help you avoid withdrawal symptoms stemming from lowering your intake of carbs and sugar.

Comparing Your Progress to Others

This is a trap that's hard to avoid falling into. People's bodies are different, so your progress has nothing to do with the progress of anyone else. Don't let yourself get discouraged if you aren't progressing as rapidly as someone else, because this discouragement can zap your will to continue the diet. Weight loss in itself is a tricky concept. It depends on a lot of factors like your age, sex, activity level, previous weight loss, and health issues. How much or how fast someone on the keto diet lost weight is not necessarily going to be the same equivalent as for you. Every body type is individually different, and every person's meals, metabolism, and lifestyle play a part in their weight loss. Don't focus on others, focus on yourself! Be sure that you are following your diet, counting your carbohydrates, preparing and eating healthy meals, managing your stress levels, and exercising to ensure your body is in a state of ketosis and burning fat. Motivate yourself and stay positive about the journey you're on. You can do it!

Allowing Setbacks in Your Progress to Impede Further Progress

Hey, we all blow it sometime, falling prey to temptation. Shake it off and accept the fact that you aren't perfect. Is anyone? Just dust yourself off and get back on track.

Not Fasting at All

Occasionally, your body needs a break from eating. Sometimes your body will drop hints that it needs a break; maybe you'll lose your appetite or get sick, which can be signs you need to fast a day or two. Fasting can also aid in establishing or re-establishing a ketosis state.

Not Getting Proper Exercise

Health expert unanimously agree that proper exercise is beneficial for your body. This doesn't necessarily mean running a marathon or taking up weight-lifting. Exercise programs should be entered gradually; extremes should be avoided. A couple short, relaxed walks every day might be all the exercise you need at the beginning. Then you can gradually start working your way to a more complete regimen.

Not drinking enough water

As we mentioned above, when you are on the keto diet, you are going to lose a lot of water weight first. That means you need to stay hydrated with plenty of fluids and electrolytes to ensure your body doesn't become dehydrated. If you exercise or live in a warmer climate, then it's especially important that you drink even more water. With keto, you need to cut out the sodas from your diet and substitute it with water instead. Sparkling water is a great alternative to still get that fizz!

Living a sedentary lifestyle

As we mentioned above, exercise and an active lifestyle is part of the formula to lose weight. If you're only changing your diet and not making the adjustments to your routine to include some physical activity, you will not properly gain the benefits of the keto diet. Try and incorporate some light aerobic activity into your day like walking or jogging for a quick 15-20 minutes. There are plenty of gym classes or workouts you can join for beginners. It's not about how hard you work out, but at least incorporating a work out into your lifestyle so your body has the chance to burn off the fat you have stored.

You're not introducing a variety of foods to your diet

There are restrictions on the keto diet, but there's also a whole array of foods that you can eat and should include in your diet! If you're eating the same things for every meal and not experimenting enough, you will feel stifled and get tired of the diet and might even have cheat meals or end up quitting. It can be tough if you're a picky eater but try and experiment with the ingredients you do like to make new recipes. Try new foods and vegetables, and whip up some fat bombs that make for tasty snacks. There are so many varieties of snacks - sweet, savory, chocolate, or full of meat and cheese! Have a variety of favorites so you aren't bored of the diet and constrained by the meal choices.

Not Knowing Your Macros

While calories count, your macros are more important when you follow the ketogenic diet. You can use a ketogenic diet calculator to figure out if you are following the recommended amounts of macros.

Avoiding Fiber

Vegetables especially the non-starchy types will always have a place in this diet. Vegetables like bell peppers, zucchini, cauliflower, and broccoli are not only rich with micronutrients but they also contain a lot of fiber that will help regulate the absorption in your stomach.

Not Dealing with Stress

Stress can affect your weight loss because it increases your cortisol levels. To cope up with the production of such hormone, the fat-burning mechanism of your body is affected, and it also increases your cravings for sugary foods. There are many ways for you to deal with stress and these include exercising, music therapy, or taking in supplements.

Eating Too Many Nuts

While nuts are great snacks for keto dieters, too many of them will kick you out of ketosis. Nuts contain high amounts of calories. For instance, 100 grams of almonds is equivalent to 700 kcal and more than 70 grams of fat that is too much for people who want to lose weight. This does not mean that you have to avoid consumption of nuts. What you can do is to reduce your total intake to a few grams.

Eating Too Much Dairy

Dairy products contain a type of protein that can lead to spikes in the insulin level. So, cut back on high-protein dairy such as cheese and yogurt. You can keep both cream and butter because they are low in that particular protein.

Eating Products that Are Labeled "Low Carb"

It is very easy to be deceived especially if the product comes with the label "low carb." The thing is that products that are labeled as such contain a lot of additives that are not good for the health.

Drinking Bulletproof Coffee

Now this keto mistake caught me off guard. I have encountered bulletproof coffee when While it can drive ketosis, I believe that bulletproof coffee has very low nutrients.

Not Planning Your Meals

When you fail to plan, then you plan to fail. Not planning your diet can easily kick you out of ketosis. Planning your meals in advance is really helpful so that you avoid excessive snacking or getting involved in binging accidents. While it is impractical to keep track of your diet forever, you can do meal prepping so that it omits the need for you to eat anything randomly.

Not Getting Enough Exercise

Not getting enough exercise is counterproductive for the keto diet. Choose the right type of exercise depending on your goals. For you to reap the most health benefits of exercise, you can do light cardio exercises as it is good for both the mind and heart. Doing weight training and high-intensity workout can also build your muscles. On the other hand, post-workout nutrition is also very important to help you succeed with the ketogenic diet. Make sure that you avoid eating foods that are high in fat exercising.

Having Cheat Meals

A part of you might be telling yourself to go and grab a burger after a week of dieting because you deserve a reward. But let me tell you that having a cheat day can kick your body out of ketosis, which is something that you worked hard for in such a long time. It is a counterproductive move for your diet.

CHAPTER 12: TIPS TO EMBRACE A KETO LIFESTYLE

Before deciding to embark on a keto-friendly diet, there are some steps you should take first. These tips are a great way to help you start the diet and to ensure you will succeed in losing weight and becoming healthier.

Stick to 30-100 grams of net carbs per day.

By "net carbs," we mean the total carbohydrate intake minus the amount of fiber. Yes, fiber is a type of carb. But fiber passes through the digestive system without being digested or used, so you don't need to count it toward your total carbs. So, just subtract the grams of fiber from the total grams of carbs.

This tip allows you to add more high-fiber vegetables to your diet without throwing off your ratio of fats to carbs and protein. It also allows you to feel fuller at the table while eating fewer calories. Not all vegetables are labeled for fiber content, but you get get that info online at various nutrition-counting sites like SELF Nutrition Data.

Determine a calorie level that's right for you.

Not everyone has the same rate of metabolism or the same nutritional needs, so a little tinkering is usually necessary until you get things right.

Basically, you're shooting for just enough calories to satisfy your hunger and keep your energy levels up. Too few calories will leave you feeling tired, and too many will prevent you from losing as much weight.

But remember that anytime you make a significant change in your diet, it will throw your system off a bit at first, so you'll probably need to tinker with your calorie levels at first, until your body adapts to the changes.

Clean Out the Cupboards

Time to give your kitchen a makeover! Ridding your cupboards, fridge, and freezer of carbs, fruits, and sugars is the best beginner tip for starting the Ketogenic Diet. You're able to give yourself a clean slate and start fresh with new foods that actually work with your body to change how your organs process foods.

All the rest must go. If you feel guilty about throwing out perfectly good food, then call up a friend or family member and bring it over to them. You can donate canned beans and boxed pastas or grains to your local food bank as well.

Create a New Keto Grocery List

Along with cleaning out your kitchen, you'll want to throw out your old grocery shopping lists, too. Those lists probably include your former cupboard staples like sandwich bread, crackers, hot dog buns, and burger buns.

But, now you're going to creating a new Keto Diet friendly grocery list.

Stock up Your Keto Kitchen

If you were thinking that many Keto Diet ingredients are expensive and hard to find, then think again. You'll mostly be purchasing produce, meats, dairy, and some condiments, so the price will be similar or perhaps even less than your current grocery bill. That's because the Keto Diet uses all natural foods!

Plan Out Your First Week's Worth of Meals

With your kitchen fully stocked with Keto ingredients to make plenty of dishes, it's time to plan out your very first seven days of meals. Have you ever meal planned before? Many don't because it seems like just one more thing to add to your busy to-do list.

Meal plans might seem to be more work than you're worth, but they're actually the number one secret to not only getting started on a new diet, but making it stick. Planning meals saves you money and time throughout the week, and, if you have a family and are cooking for more than just yourself, it answers that daily question, "What's for dinner?"

You might also want to add certain cooking notes and plan out how you're going to make the meals, too.

What's Your Schedule?

While you're planning out your meals, think of how the Keto Diet can realistically fit into your weekly schedule. You'll want easy morning recipes that are simple to make, work snacks and lunches you can pack and take to your job, simple dinners that don't take long to prepare after work, and a couple of sweet treats to give you some indulgence in the evening. All of this should be accomplished with Keto ingredients, too.

You might also want to think about the times you get hungry during the day. Are you a desk snack? A TV-and-munchies eater? We're not trying to drastically eliminate all of your secret snacking times, but it is important to keep in mind that you're used to reaching for carb snacks like cookies, crackers, and chips.

You're going to want to replace those carb snacks with the Keto Diet ones, which are listed as part of the grocery store ingredients and in the recipes. Snack times do strike us all, and it helps to have Keto fat bombs in the fridge as a pick-me-up. Oh, you don't know what a fat bomb is? You are in for a treat!

You're not only planning out your meals, you're also planning out how to live without carbs! Make the Keto Diet work with your schedule, so that you're not reaching for 'convenience carbs.' Instead, you're reaching for 'fast fats!'

Focus on Eating What You Love

It can be all too easy and tempting to fall into the mindset that "diets equal deprivation." It's called a diet, so it must be hardcore, prevent you from eating your favorite foods, and basically be a way to torture yourself, right? This Keto Diet in particular sounds difficult, because there's no carbs!

Well, not in this case! The Keto Diet doesn't have carbs, that's true, but carbs only make up a single portion of your diet. There's an entire supermarket of flavor waiting for you outside of the bakery section and the potato chip aisle.

Fill your kitchen with your favorite flavors and foods. You'll enjoy the cheeses, butters and oils, cream, milk, eggs, meats, fresh veggies, herbs and spices, and nuts that are included on the Keto Diet.

The more you focus on eating what you love, the better the Keto Diet will be overall for you.

Try Different Flavor Combinations

The Keto Diet will work best for you if it tastes good! One of the little known secrets to becoming a great cook is to understand and work with different flavor combinations. Every cuisine on the planet has its own specific group of flavors. After you purchase those ingredients, you can use those flavors to marinade meat, create a cheese or egg dish, and spice up fresh veggies.

Use Keto Sticks or Strips

Since you're measuring ketosis on the Keto Diet, you want to have a scientific way to check that your liver is breaking down fat properly to produce ketones. You can find special ketone strips or sticks on Amazon, at Walmart, and at other major retailers. These sticks are meant for beginners and can be very helpful. They measure your urine.

When you get your keto sticks, open them up. Hold the keto stick in your urine stream for a few seconds and then set it on a clean paper towel. Within about 10-15 seconds, you'll see the strip change color. Ketone urine sticks are usually measured on the red spectrum. If it shows up light pink, that means you're low in ketone production. The darker the red, the more in ketosis you are! Deep ketosis is in the optimal weight loss range.

As you get more comfortable and familiar with the diet, you'll want to invest in measuring your ketones with special breath meters and the more expensive but very accurate blood meter.

Monitor any side effects you might experience during the early stages of the diet.

People react differently to changes in diet. Symptoms might include dizziness, fatigue, quickening heart rate and shortness of breath. If any of these symptoms occur, it's probably a good idea to avoid strenuous activity, though light exercise is probably fine and might well help alleviate the symptoms. If these symptoms seem serious or if they persist for more than a few days, it's probably a good idea to talk to your doctor.

Monitoring side effects is especially important for diabetics and other people with insulin problems who might be prone to ketoacidosis, a dangerous condition.

Test your ketone levels and compare the results to your meal choices.

The main idea behind this diet is to raise the level of ketones in your bloodstream, ensuring that you're entering ketosis and burning fat instead of glucose. To keep track of this, you should test your ketone levels daily and compare them to what you ate that day. This will give you graphic evidence of what's going on in your body so that you can make the proper choices to regulate your diet. In particular, it will help in determining the ideal level of carbs you should be eating.

Decrease the stress factors in your life. A stressful lifestyle can actually cause you to gain weight and send false hunger signals to your body. If you're going to be making the change to a keto lifestyle, it's important you are in the right period of your life to make the changes with enthusiasm. If you're going through a stressful patch, then maybe delay the diet until you feel more at calm with your life. If you still want to start the keto diet, that's great too, but be sure you are taking time to decompress from the stress of your day. Whether it's exercising, yoga, meditation, or ensuring you have a good night's sleep, you want to take some personal time to relax from a stressful lifestyle so your body can follow through on the demands of a keto diet.

Stay hydrated

Staying hydrated is an important factor to overall health no matter what diet you are on. During a keto diet, it's even more important at the start of your diet because your body first excretes water weight when you switch to a low carb lifestyle. To combat this, it's important you have a habit of drinking enough water to avoid dehydration. That number needs to be increased if the temperature is hotter or if you've been exercising. So if you're going to start keto, it's a great idea to already adjust to drinking enough water. Keep a water bottle with you and keep it visible at all times to remind yourself to take a few sips.

Count your carbs.

If you're serious about following a keto lifestyle, you will have to count your macros and your carbohydrates when you first begin, as you and your appetite get adjusted to what you can and cannot eat. To help yourself out, start counting carbohydrates in your normal diet to get an idea of just how much you will have to restrict yourself. Don't forget those hidden carbs! Things like fruit, milk, and condiments also have carbs that should be counted. Look at the nutrition facts and be consciously aware of what you're eating. You want to calculate net carbs: Total carbs - Fiber = Net Carbs. You want to try and naturally lower your carbohydrates so you can drop down even lower when you're on the keto diet. There are tons of apps you can download to help you!

Get rid of those carbs!

Look, the truth of the matter is, you're going to keep eating what you have access to. If you keep carbohydrates in stock, you're going to keep having them simply because they're there. So to begin your keto diet, go ahead and clear out all the carbohydrates you have from your pantry. Bread, pasta, cereal, snacks, candy, rice, processed snacks... it sounds drastic and you might be aghast at how much empty space you have! But that's space you can fill up with healthy ingredients that will make up your keto lifestyle.

Keep keto friendly snacks on hand.

This is a common pitfall for people who are embarking on the keto diet. They may meticulously plan out their keto friendly meals, but if a craving hits, and they satisfy it with an unhealthy snack... there goes your macro count for the day! To combat this, finish up all those unhealthy snacks in your pantry and fill it up with the healthy stuff! Try having more protein like bacon slices, beef jerky, and eggs. Fat bombs are also very simple recipes you can make to get a taste of what type of snacks you should be eating.

Be prepared for when you're eating out.

When you first start the keto diet, it can seem overwhelming when you're at a restaurant trying to decide what is keto friendly and what isn't. But it gets easier if you know exactly what to ask for! Make sure you have your lists of approved keto foods and don't hesitate to ask for substitutes of sides in a meal. For breakfast, eggs and bacon is a great meal and very filling! Say no to the pancakes or waffles and see if there's a healthy omelet with veggies you have can have instead. Lunch will always have a salad option for you. Be sure you ask for simple vinegar or olive oil dressing instead of one loaded with sugar! And for dinner, you can focus on protein by ordering a nice steak or salmon. For a side, order a serving of vegetables on the keto list like broccoli or cauliflower instead of potatoes or French fries.

Start exercising.

If you're not already living an active lifestyle, it's important that you transition to one if you want to see weight loss results on a keto lifestyle. Coupled with the healthy diet, you also need exercise to get rid of the glucose molecules your body has stored as fat. Try and go to the gym a few times a week, or at least incorporate exercises like jogging or walking for a quick 15 to 20 minutes every day. You don't have to exercise every day, but a combination of strength training and aerobic workouts can induce weight loss much quicker than a sedentary lifestyle. Look up beginner workouts and incorporate a training schedule into your week! Grab a workout buddy to have extra motivation!

Cut the soda and sugar from your diet. Just like we mentioned above with carbohydrates, it's also important that you're aware of how much sugar you're ingesting throughout the day. Whether it's just a spoon or two in your morning coffee, a sweet treat at lunch, or a handful of cookies before bed, all of that sugar you're going to cut from your lifestyle when you go keto. Start cutting back on that now. Diet soda is also detrimental to the keto diet because it uses sugar substitutes that send signals to your body as if sugar is entering your bloodstream. This increases your blood sugar levels and can produce extra fat molecules. No more diet sodas! Try sparkling water instead!

Invest in a food scale or measuring tools. As a keto beginner, weighing the food you eat and being aware of portion sizes is going to be key. Buy a food scale if you don't have one so that way you feel confident about portion sizes when trying new recipes. Also, make sure you have proper measuring spoons and cups. There's a big difference between one tablespoon of almond butter and two tablespoons - that's an extra 200 calories and as much as 7 carbohydrates you'd be gaining that you don't need! Spoons/cups and food scales are relatively inexpensive and you should find a handy space for them in your kitchen since you will be frequently using them in the beginning as you get used to serving sizes.

Educate yourself on a keto diet! Last but not least, if you're going to be embarking on a keto lifestyle, it's important you know exactly what you're getting into. Taking the time to read the appropriate literature (like this book!) is a great start, as well as listening to podcasts or viewing videos of people who successfully live the keto lifestyle. Find printable that show which foods are on the keto-friendly list so you become familiar when you are shopping or eating out. The more familiar you are, the more confident you'll feel about your lifestyle choices.

CHAPTER 13: YOUR 14 DAY MEAL PLAN

Day 1

   Breakfast: Gluten-Free, Keto Coconut Bread

   Lunch: Shrimp Tuscany

   Snack: Simplest wraps ever

   Dinner: Beefy Pizza

   Smoothie: Keto Green Smoothie

Day 2

   Breakfast: Baked Brussels Sprout with Garlic

   Lunch: Pork Salad

   Snack: Peaches and Creamy Cheese

   Dinner: Bacon Cheeseburger Casserole

   Smoothie: Keto All in One Smoothie

Day 3

   Breakfast: Spinach Rolls

   Lunch: Shrimp in Tuscan Cream Sauce

   Snack: The Hodge Podge Grab Bag

   Dinner: Pan-Fried Chops

   Smoothie: Pumpkin Protein Smoothie

Day 4

   Breakfast: Low-Carb Breakfast Balls

   Lunch: Almond Pesto Salmon

   Snack: Heavenly mushrooms

   Dinner: Balsamic Beef Roast

   Smoothie: Pumpkin Protein Smoothie

Day 5

Breakfast: Keto Muffins with Chicken

Lunch: Salmon and Potato Salad

Snack: Sunrise Kabobs

Dinner: Bacon & BBQ Cheeseburger Waffles

Smoothie: Healthy Green Smoothie

Day 6

Breakfast: Borecole with Curry

Lunch: Mediterranean Tuna

Snack: Fishy Jerky

Dinner: Cumin Spiced Beef Wraps

Smoothie: Spinach Cucumber Smoothie

Day 7

Breakfast: Eggs on Sour Cream

Lunch: Smoked Salmon

Snack: Savory Wraps

Dinner: Ground Beef Stir Fry

Smoothie: Spinach Peanut Butter Smoothie

Day 8

Breakfast: Zucchini in Yogurt

Lunch: Salmon Fishcakes

Snack: Beef and Cheese

Dinner: Chicken Fried Pork Chops

Smoothie: Choco Fat Bomb Smoothie

Day 9

Breakfast: Gluten-Free, Keto Coconut Bread

Lunch: Omega-3 Rich Salmon Soup

Snack: Turkey Tugs

Dinner: Parmesan Crusted Pork Chops

Smoothie: Avocado Smoothie

Day 10

Breakfast: Baked Brussels Sprout with Garlic

Lunch: chili lime cod

Snack: Hard Boiled Power Balls

Dinner: Beef Burritos

Smoothie: Raspberry Smoothie

Day 11

Breakfast: Mini Chocolate Cakes

Lunch: Cauliflower Taboule Salad

Snack: Simplest wraps ever

Dinner: Pork Salad

Smoothie: Spinach Cucumber Smoothie

Day 12

Breakfast: Vanilla Bean Cheesecake

Lunch: Vegetarian Club Salad

Snack: Peaches and Creamy Cheese

Dinner: Crispy Pork Salad

Smoothie: Keto Green Smoothie

Day 13

Breakfast: Raspberry Cookies

Lunch: Thai Pork Salad

Snack: The Hodge Podge Grab Bag

Dinner: Cauliflower Taboule Salad

Smoothie: Pumpkin Protein Smoothie

Day 14

Breakfast: Easy Almond Bars

Lunch: Caprese Salad

Snack: Heavenly mushrooms

Dinner: Bistro Steak Salad with Horseradish Dressing

Smoothie: Raspberry Smoothie

CHAPTER 14: 14 DAY SHOPPING LIST

Week 1

Shopping list

- 20 eggs
- 2 oz. baking powder
- 2 oz. of coconut flour
- 4 oz. butter
- 1 oz. salt
- Baby kale (.25 c.)
- 5 Oz. Tomatoes
- 2 Oz. Parmesan
- 3 oz. Dried basil
- 5 garlic cloves
- 5 c. Whole milk
- 1 c. Cream cheese
- 6 lb. shrimp
- ¼ oz. shredded cheddar cheese
- 7 lb. pork chops
- 1 large green lettuce leaf
- 14 oz. of Brussels sprout
- 1 oz. ground pork rinds
- 30 oz. ground beef
- 3 oz. frozen strawberries
- 2 oz. fresh baby spinach
- 1 can coconut milk

- 3 oz. of chili pepper
- 10 oz. olive oil
- 3 oz. pepperoni slices
- 6 oz. Pizza sauce
- 4 oz. mozzarella cheese
- 5 lb Pork belly slices
- 3 oz. White wine vinegar
- 3 oz. Mustard
- 2 oz. liquid stevia
- 3 oz. vanilla extract
- 5 oz. fresh mint leaves
- 5 oz. unsweetened coconut milk
- 3 oz. pistachio
- 6 avocadoes

Week 2

Shopping list

- 4 oz. heavy cream
- 1 oz. baking cocoa
- 2 oz. baking powder
- 5 oz. Splenda
- 4 oz. vanilla
- 8 oz. zucchini
- 7 oz. cup of yogurt
- 3 oz. Oregano
- 24 eggs
- 14 oz. cup almond flour

- 2 oz. baking powder
- 3 oz. baking soda
- 5 oz. unsweetened almond milk
- 4 oz. pumpkin pie spice
- 5 lb. Pork belly slices
- 8 oz. whole almonds
- 4 oz. mozzarella cheese stick
- 9 oz. peanuts
- 10 oz. large white mushrooms
- 12 lb.rib-eye steak
- 4 oz. Pepper
- 6 oz. Salt
- 2.1 oz. small red onion
- 7 oz. bag romaine salad greens
- 19 oz. bacon
- 2 oz. sliced radishes
- 1 oz. cherry tomatoes
- 14 oz. horseradish
- 13 oz. mayonnaise
- 4 oz. almond butter
- 5 oz. Swerve
- 4 oz. raw almonds
- 6 oz. raspberry extract
- 23 lb. turkey breast slices
- 4 oz. cheddar cheese
- 7 oz. frozen raspberries
- 4 oz. raspberry extract
- 2 oz. cocoa powder

- 6 avocadoes
- 7 oz. unsweetened almond milk
- 3 oz. Cauliflower florets
- 4 oz. Parsley
- 5 oz. mint leaves
- 7 oz. tomatoes
- 4 oz. cucumbers
- 14 oz. Lemon juice
- 4 oz. Olive oil

CHAPTER 15: KETO BREAKFAST RECIPES

1. Gluten-Free, Keto Coconut Bread

Preparing time: 10 minutes

Serves: 6

Ingredients:

- 2 eggs
- 1 teaspoon of baking powder
- 2 tbsp. of coconut flour
- 2 teaspoons of butter
- 1 teaspoon of salt

Directions:

1. Whisk eggs and salt them.
2. Mix them with flour and baking powder.
3. Pour mixture into 2 ceramic cups.
4. Cook them in a microwave for 2 minutes at max heat.
5. Enjoy your ideal fast ketogenic bread!

Nutritional information Per Serving (Calories 132 | Total Fats 6.9g | Net Carbs: 7g | Protein 3.2g |Fiber: 7.3g)

2. Baked Brussels Sprout with Garlic

Preparing time: 35 minutes

Serves: 6

Ingredients

- 14 oz. of Brussels sprout
- 1 tbsp. of powdered garlic
- ½ teaspoon of chili pepper
- 4 tbsp. of olive oil
- Pinch of salt

Directions:

1. Cook Brussels sprout in boiling water for 2 minutes.
2. Strain the water, add powdered garlic and pepper.
3. Sprinkle everything with olive oil and add salt.
4. Pour mixture into a casserole dish to bake for 25 minutes at 220 F.

Nutritional information Per Serving (Calories 132 | Total Fats 6.9g | Net Carbs: 7g | Protein 3.2g |Fiber: 7.3g)

3. Spinach Rolls

Preparing time: 30 minutes

Serves: 6

Ingredients:

- 7 oz. of white meat (cut into small cubes)
- 1 cup of spinach
- 4 eggs
- 7 oz. of cream cheese
- 1 tbsp. of sesame seeds
- ½ teaspoon of sodium bicarbonate 4 tbsp. of flour

Directions:

1. Cook spinach and meat in water. (Separately)
2. Whish 3 eggs with 4 tbsp. of flour, sodium, salt, 2 tbsp. of cheese, and ½ cup of cooked spinach.
3. Mix them well and then put them to bake at 250 F for 10 minutes.
4. In a meanwhile, dissolve a pinch of salt in water. Add ½ cup of cooked spinach, meat and 1 egg. Cook the mixture in a cooking pot until meat is done.
5. Cut baked dough into smaller sizes, fill them with cooked mixture and roll.
6. Enjoy!

Nutritional information Per Serving (Calories 132 | Total Fats 6.9g | Net Carbs: 7g | Protein 3.2g |Fiber: 7.3g)

4. Low-Carb Breakfast Balls

Preparing time: 25 minutes

Serves: 6

Ingredients:

- 7 oz. of chicken meat
- 3 oz. of cheese
- 1 tbsp. of sour cream
- 2 tbsp. of mayonnaise
- ½ cup of olives (ground)
- Cheese for rolling

Directions:

1. Cook chicken meat in water. When it is done, cut it into very tiny pieces or grind it.
2. Combine meat with cheese, sour cream and mayonnaise.
3. Make small balls out of the mixture and then roll them into the cheese.
4. Serve and enjoy!

Nutritional information Per Serving (Calories 132 | Total Fats 6.9g | Net Carbs: 7g | Protein 3.2g |Fiber: 7.3g)

5. Keto Muffins with Chicken

Preparing time: 50 minutes

Serves: 6

Ingredients:

- 4 oz. of chicken fillets
- 2 eggs
- 3 teaspoons of cheese
- 6 teaspoons of oat flakes
- Spices to taste

Directions:

1. Cut fillets into tiny pieces.
2. Separate egg yolks from egg whites.
3. Combine egg yolk with cheese, meat, flakes, and spices.
4. Blend whites into dense cream.
5. Gradually, join 2 mixtures together.
6. Pour resulting mixture into muffin molds and bake for 20 minutes at 250 F.

Nutritional information Per Serving (Calories 132 | Total Fats 6.9g | Net Carbs: 7g | Protein 3.2g |Fiber: 7.3g)

6. Borecole with Curry

Preparing time: 30 minutes

Serves: 6

Ingredients:

- 2 eggs
- 10 oz. of borecole
- Salt, pepper to taste
- 1 tbsp. of powdered curry

Directions:

1. Wash borecole and cut it thinly. Cook it in water for 10 minutes, so it becomes soft.
2. Whisk eggs with spices. Mix well.
3. Soak borecole into prepared eggs mixture and put it on an oiled baking tray.
4. Bake for 15 minutes at 300 F.

Nutritional information Per Serving (Calories 132 | Total Fats 6.9g | Net Carbs: 7g | Protein 3.2g |Fiber: 7.3g)

7. Eggs on Sour Cream

Preparing time: 35 minutes

Serves: 6

Ingredients

- 6 eggs
- 1 cup of sour cream
- 1 tbsp. of parsley
- 1 tbsp. of butter
- Salt to taste

Directions:

1. Spread sour cream over casserole dish equally.
2. Make 6 holes in the sour cream mixture and pour the egg into each one.
3. Add salt and parsley. Bake for 15 minutes at 250 F.

Nutritional information Per Serving (Calories 132 | Total Fats 6.9g | Net Carbs: 7g | Protein 3.2g |Fiber: 7.3g)

8. Zucchini in Yogurt

Preparing time: 15 minutes

Serves: 6

Ingredients:

- 1 zucchini
- 1 cup of yogurt
- Salt, pepper, and oregano to taste

Directions:

1. Cut zucchinis into circles. Pour salt over them and let them sit for 5 minutes.
2. Strain the water, and sauté zucchini circles in a frying pan. (Without oil)
3. Pour yogurt over zucchini and serve!

Nutritional information Per Serving (Calories 132 | Total Fats 6.9g | Net Carbs: 7g | Protein 3.2g |Fiber: 7.3g)

9. Gluten-Free, Keto Coconut Bread

Preparing time: 10 minutes

Serves: 6

Ingredients:

- 2 eggs
- 1 teaspoon of baking powder
- 2 tbsp. of coconut flour
- 2 teaspoons of butter
- 1 teaspoon of salt

Directions:

Whisk eggs and salt them.

Mix them with flour and baking powder.

Pour mixture into 2 ceramic cups.

Cook them in a microwave for 2 minutes at max heat.

Enjoy your ideal fast ketogenic bread!

Nutritional information Per Serving (Calories 132 | Total Fats 6.9g | Net Carbs: 7g | Protein 3.2g |Fiber: 7.3g)

10.   Baked Brussels Sprout with Garlic

Preparing time: 35 minutes

Serves: 6

Ingredients:

- 14 oz. of Brussels sprout
- 1 tbsp. of powdered garlic
- ½ teaspoon of chili pepper
- 4 tbsp. of olive oil
- Pinch of salt

Directions:

5. Cook Brussels sprout in boiling water for 2 minutes.
6. Strain the water, add powdered garlic and pepper.
7. Sprinkle everything with olive oil and add salt.
8. Pour mixture into a casserole dish to bake for 25 minutes at 220 F.

Nutritional information Per Serving (Calories 132 | Total Fats 6.9g | Net Carbs: 7g | Protein 3.2g |Fiber: 7.3g)

CHAPTER 16: KETO SMOOTHIES

11.　Keto Green Smoothie

Time: 10 minutes

Serve: 1

Ingredients:

- ½ cup ice cubes
- ½ cup water
- 5 drops liquid stevia
- 1 tsp vanilla extract
- 4 fresh mint leaves
- ½ cup egg whites
- ¼ cup spinach
- ¼ cup unsweetened coconut milk
- 2 tbsp pistachio
- 1 avocado

Directions:

1. Add all ingredients into the blender and blend until smooth and creamy.

2. Serve immediately and enjoy.

Nutritional Value (Amount per Serving): Calories 328 Fat 23.3 g Carbohydrates 12.5 g Sugar 3.9 g Protein 18.3 g Cholesterol 0 mg

12. Keto All in One Smoothie

Time: 5 minutes

Serve: 2

Ingredients:

- ½ ice cubes
- 1 tbsp coconut oil
- 2 tbsp heavy cream
- 1 cup unsweetened almond milk
- 1 tsp chia seeds
- 4 raspberries
- 4 walnuts
- 1 cup spinach

Directions:

1. Add all ingredients into the blender and blend until everything is well combined.
2. Serve immediately and enjoy.

Nutritional Value (Amount per Serving): Calories 188, Fat 17.1 g Carbohydrates 7.3 g Sugar 1.7 g Protein 2.5 g Cholesterol 20 mg

13. Pumpkin Protein Smoothie

Preparing time: 10 minutes

Serves: 6

Ingredients:

- ½ cup ice cubes
- 5 drops liquid stevia
- 1 tsp pumpkin pie spice
- ¼ tsp ground cinnamon
- 1 tbsp unsweetened cocoa powder
- 1 tbsp ground flax seed
- ½ cup cottage cheese
- ½ cup unsweetened almond milk
- ¼ cup pumpkin puree

Directions:

1. Add all ingredients into the blender and blend until smooth and well combined.

2. Serve immediately and enjoy.

Nutritional Value (Amount per Serving): Calories 179 Fat 6.2 g Carbohydrates 14 g Sugar 5 g Protein 17.7 g Cholesterol 5 mg

THE KETO DIET FOR BEGINNERS

14.　Green Protein Smoothie

Time: 5 minutes

Serve: 2

Ingredients:

- ½ cup egg whites
- 1 cup frozen strawberries
- 2 cups fresh baby spinach
- 1 can coconut milk
- 5 drops liquid stevia

Directions:

1. Add all ingredients into the blender and blend until smooth and creamy.
2. Serve immediately and enjoy.

Nutritional Value (Amount per Serving): Calories 126 Fat 6.2 g Carbohydrates 9.5 g Sugar 5 g Protein 8.2 g Cholesterol 0 mg

15. Healthy Green Smoothie

Preparing time: 10 minutes

Serve: 1

Ingredients:

- 1/2 scoop protein powder
- 1/4 avocado, chopped
- 1/2 cup cucumber, chopped
- 1/2 tsp liquid stevia
- 1/4 cup cream
- 1/2 cup coconut milk
- 4 ice cubes

Directions:

1. Add all ingredients into the blender and blend until smooth.
2. Serve and enjoy.

Nutritional Value (Amount per Serving): Calories 271 Fat 20.1 g Carbohydrates 11.4 g Sugar 2.8 g Protein 13.6 g Cholesterol 44 mg

16. Spinach Cucumber Smoothie

Time: 5 minutes

Serve: 1

Ingredients:

- 1 tbsp MCT oil
- ¼ tsp xanthan gum
- 10 drops liquid stevia
- 1 cup unsweetened coconut milk
- ½ cup ice cubes
- 2.3 oz cucumber, peeled and diced
- 2 cups spinach

Directions:

1. Add all ingredients into the blender and blend until smooth and creamy.
2. Serve immediately and enjoy.

Nutritional Value (Amount per Serving): Calories 172 Fat 18.3 g Carbohydrates 7.4 g Sugar 1.3 g Protein 2.1 g Cholesterol 0 mg

17.   Spinach Peanut Butter Smoothie

Time: 5 minutes

Serve: **1**

Ingredients:

- 2 tbsp peanut butter
- 1 scoop chocolate protein powder
- 1 cup fresh spinach
- ¾ cup unsweetened almond milk

Directions:

1. Add all ingredients into the blender and blend until smooth.
2. Serve immediately and enjoy.

Nutritional Value (Amount per Serving): Calories 280 Fat 19.6 g Carbohydrates 10.9 g Sugar 4.1 g Protein 19.6 g Cholesterol 20 mg

18.   Choco Fat Bomb Smoothie

Preparing time: 10 minutes

Serves: 6

Ingredients:

- 2.5 oz frozen avocado pieces
- ½ cup ice cubes
- 1 cup almond milk S
- 1 tbsp cocoa powder
- 1 scoop perfect keto chocolate collagen

Directions:

1. Add all ingredients into the blender and blend until completely smooth and creamy.
2. Serve immediately and enjoy.

Nutritional Value (Amount per Serving): Calories 326 Fat 18.7 g Carbohydrates 12.3 g Sugar 0.4 g Protein 33.4 g Cholesterol 7 mg

19. Avocado Smoothie

Preparing time: 5 minutes

Serves: 6

Ingredients:

- 2 tbsp cocoa powder
- 4 oz vanilla Greek yogurt
- ½ avocado
- 3 tbsp unsweetened almond milk

Directions:

1. Add all ingredients into the blender and blend until smooth and creamy.
2. Serve and enjoy.

Nutritional Value (Amount per Serving): Calories 78 Fat 4.6 g Carbohydrates 9.4 g Sugar 1.6 g Protein 4.9 g Cholesterol 1 mg

20.   Raspberry Smoothie

Preparing time: 5 minutes

Serves: 6

Ingredients:

- 1/3 cup frozen raspberries
- 1/8 tsp raspberry extract
- 1 tbsp. swerve
- 1 tbsp. cocoa powder
- ½ avocado
- 1 ¼ cup unsweetened almond milk

Directions:

1. Add all ingredients into the blender and blend until smooth and creamy.
2. Serve and enjoy.

Nutritional Value (Amount per Serving): Calories 81 Fat 2.9 g Carbohydrates 15.1 g Sugar 9.1 g Protein 1.5 g Cholesterol 0 mg

CHAPTER 17: KETO SNACKS

21. Simplest wraps ever

Preparing time:25 minutes

Serves: 2

Ingredients:

- ¼ cup shredded cheddar cheese
- 1 large green lettuce leaf
- 1 toothpick

Directions:

1. Lay out the lettuce leaf, make sure the stem is removed if you are using romaine lettuce.
2. Sprinkle the cheese in the middle of the lettuce, wrap up like you would a chicken wrap, and secure with the toothpick.

Nutritional information per serving Calories: 212 | Protein: 15g | Fat: 32.2 g | Net Carbs: 2.3 g Fiber: 4.3g

22. Peaches and Creamy Cheese

Preparing time: 20 minutes

Serves: 2

Ingredients:

- 1 medium peach
- Cottage cheese
- Stevia

Directions:

1. Using a sharp knife, carefully remove the pit from the peach. Then, thinly slice the peach into a dish.
2. Remove 1/3 of the peach and put on your plate, then keep the rest of the peach in your fridge until later.
3. Take ½ cup of the cottage cheese and spread on a dessert plate.
4. Evenly place the third of the peach across the top of the cottage cheese, and sprinkle with stevia. Serve.

Nutritional information per serving Calories: 254 | Protein: 5 g | Fat: 34 g | Net Carbs: 2 g Fiber: 6g

23. The Hodge Podge Grab Bag

Preparing time:15 minutes

Serves: 2

Ingredients:

- ¼ cup whole almonds
- 1 mozzarella cheese stick
- ¼ cup peanuts

Directions:

1. Slice the cheese stick up to make small cubes, about the same size as the almonds.
2. Place everything in a zip lock bag and that's it! One of the fastest and easiest things to grab on the run, this snack will be sure to satisfy without breaking your carb goal for the day!

Nutritional information per serving Calories: 219 | Protein: 30 g | Fat: 32 g | Net Carbs: 7 g Fiber: 7g

24. Heavenly mushrooms

Preparing time:10 minutes

Serves: 2

Ingredients:

- 4 large white mushrooms… about one cup
- ½ cup shredded cheese
- 3 ounces' cream cheese
- 1 cup cooked pork sausage

Directions:

1. Heat up the cooked pork sausage and set aside. Pull the stems off of the mushrooms, cut up the stems, and add to the pork sausage.
2. Melt the cheeses together in a pan turned on to medium high heat on the stove. Transfer to the pan with the pork sausage and mix everything together. Place all of the mushroom tops with the bottom facing up in a baking dish.
3. Stuff the stuffing into the bottoms of the mushrooms, and place the whole thing in the oven for 15 minutes, or until the white mushrooms have turned golden brown.
4. Eat hot with a fork.

Nutritional information per serving Calories: 426 | Protein: 30.8 g | Fat: 32.2 g | Net Carbs: 4.3 g Fiber: 7.3g

25. Sunrise Kabobs

Preparing time:35 minutes

Serves: 2

Ingredients:

- 1 cheddar string cheese
- 2 large strawberries
- ½ cup grape tomatoes
- Kabob stick

Directions:

1. Wash the fruit, and, taking your knife, slice the string cheese into cubes, about the same size as the grape tomatoes.
2. Arrange on your kabob stick, varying the cheese and fruit so they are all arranged nicely and not all together in a group.
3. If you want to add a bit of a Hawaiian flare to them, roast them in your oven with a bit of dried, no sugar added, coconut on top.
4. Please note that the coconut will add a few more grams of carbs to your snack, but even with those you will still stay well under 10 grams for the whole thing.
5. If you choose to roast them, roast in the oven for 10 minutes at 350 degrees F.

Nutritional information per serving Calories: 218 | Protein: 36 g | Fat: 28 g | Net Carbs: 6g Fiber: 8g

26. Fishy Jerky

Preparing time:15 minutes

Serves: 2

Ingredients:

- Salt and pepper to taste
- 6 ounces catfish

Directions:

1. Turn on your oven as low as it can go, and line a baking sheet with parchment paper. Slice the catfish thinly, and lay on the parchment paper.

2. Sprinkle with the salt and pepper, lighter on the salt as you want the fish to dry into jerky, not dry out.

3. Let dry roast in your oven for 8 hours, then pull out and test. If it is still tender, put in your oven for another 2 hours, until the catfish has become jerky.

4. You can make this in a lot bigger of a batch than just a single serving, simply store the rest in an air tight container and keep it stored in a cool place.

Nutritional information per serving Calories: 318| Protein: 30g | Fat: 29.2 g | Net Carbs: 5g Fiber: 6g

27. Savory Wraps

It is easy to make and once your guests get a taste of it, I know they will be begging you for the recipe.

Preparing time:20 minutes

Serves: 2

Ingredients:

- 5 ounces thinly sliced roast beef
- 1 celery stalk
- 3 ounces cream cheese
- Salt and pepper, to taste

Directions:

1. Soften the cream cheese in the microwave. Slice the celery into thin, horse shoe shapes, and mix in with the cream cheese.
2. Lay out the strips of roast beef, then spread with the cream cheese and celery.
3. Sprinkle with salt and pepper, then roll into wraps. Secure with a toothpick if necessary.

Nutritional information per serving Calories: 312| Protein: 30.8 g | Fat: 32.2 g | Net Carbs: 4.3 g Fiber: 7.3g

28. Beef and Cheese

It is easy to make and once your guests get a taste of it, I know they will be begging you for the recipe.

Preparing time:25 minutes

Serves: 2

Ingredients:

- 6 ounces roast beef
- 2 slices cheddar cheese

Directions:

1. Thinly cut the cheese into strips, and set aside.
2. Lay out the strips of roast beef, and lay the cheese inside.
3. Roll the beef around the cheese, and place in the microwave.
4. Melt the cheese inside the beef rolls, and enjoy with a fork.

Nutritional information per serving Calories: 164| Protein: 38g | Fat: 30g | Net Carbs: 6g Fiber: 5g

29. Turkey Tugs

Preparing time:15 minutes

Serves: 2

Ingredients:

- 3 turkey breast slices
- 1 tablespoon mayo
- 1 stick cheddar cheese
- 1 pickle

Directions:

1. Lay the turkey breast on a plate, and divide the mayo among the three. Slice the cheese into 3 thin slices and the pickle as well.
2. Lay these side by side on the turkey breast, then roll up.
3. Secure with a toothpick, if desired, and you are ready to enjoy! These are also the perfect on the go snack, all you need to do is put them in a zip lock bag and you are ready to head out the door to take on whatever your day is throwing your way.

Nutritional information per serving Calories: 160| Protein: 30.8 g | Fat: 32.2 g | Net Carbs: 4.3 g Fiber: 7.3g

30. Hard Boiled Power Balls

Preparing time:20 minutes

Serves: 2

Ingredients:

- 1 dozen eggs
- Large pot
- Water

Directions:

1. Place the eggs carefully in the pot and cover them generously with water.
2. Be careful not to crack any of them as you are doing this. Cover the eggs with cold water and place on the stove.
3. Turn the burner on to medium high heat, and bring to a boil.
4. Once the eggs are boiling, boil them for 3 minutes, then cover them and remove them from the heat.
5. Let the water cool with the eggs still in it, then run the eggs under cold water in a colander.
6. Now, you can either store them in your fridge in the shell, or, if you plan to eat them sooner, you can peel all of the shells off at once and store them that way, it is really up to you.

Nutritional information per serving Calories: 176| Protein: 39.8 g | Fat: 28.2 g | Net Carbs: 2.3 g Fiber: 4.3g

CHAPTER 18: KETO DRESSING, SALADS AND SAUCES

31. Pork Salad

Prep time: 15 minutes

Cooking time: 30 minutes

Servings: 2

Ingredients

- Sliced pear (.25)
- Blue cheese (.33 c.)
- Pork belly slices (.5 lb.)
- Olive oil (2 tsp.)
- White wine vinegar (2 Tbsp.)
- Mustard (.5 tsp.)
- Water (1 tsp.)
- Stevia (1 Tbsp.)
- Chopped walnuts (.3 c.)
- Sat (2 tsp.)
- Salad leaves (2 c.)

Instructions:

1. Cover the pork with half your oil and then cook it in the oven for 30 minutes.

2. Warm up a pan and add the stevia and water. When the stevia dissolves, add the walnuts and cook for about five minutes.

3. Take the nuts and allow them to cool. While those are cooling, chop the cheese and pear into smaller bits.

4. To make the dressing, add the oil, vinegar, and mustard to a bowl.

5. Take the pork out of the oven and slice into smaller bits. Toss the salad with the dressing before adding the rest of the ingredients and serving.

Nutritional Information: Calories: 567 Fats: 55g Carbs: 5g Protein: 13g

32. Salmon and Potato Salad

Prep time: 10 minutes

Cooking time: 25 minutes

Servings: 6

Ingredients

- Chopped parsley (1 Tbsp.)
- Salmon (6 oz.)
- Chopped onion (1)
- Olive oil (1 Tbsp.)
- Baking potatoes (3)

Directions:

1. Boil the potatoes and eggs together until done. While those are boiling, heat up some oil in a pan and fry the onions.
2. Place the salmon slices into a dish and put the onions on top.
3. Top with the eggs and he potatoes and sprinkle the parsley on top before serving.

Nutritional Information: Calories: 370 Fat: 30g Carbs: 10g Protein: 15g

33. Crispy Pork Salad

Prep time: 10 minutes

Cooking time: 5 minutes

Servings: 2

Ingredients for the Dish

- ½ lb. of pork belly slices
- 1/3 cup of blue cheese
- ¼ of a pear, sliced
- 2 cups of salad leave of your choice (rocket goes well with pear…)
- 2 tsp of salt
- 1/3 cup of chopped walnuts
- 1 tbsp. of stevia
- 1 tsp of water
- ½ tsp of Dijon mustard
- ½ tsp of any whole grain mustard for the dressing
- 2 tbsp. of white wine vinegar
- 2 tsp of olive oil

Instructions:

1. Prepare all ingredients in advance, and store in glass containers. If packing your lunch, the morning of, assemble your salad, in a container and put the dressing in a separate container.
2. Measure out the ingredients in advance.
3. Do any chopping; a squeeze of lemon juice will help the pear chunks to stay crisp.
4. Making the Dish

5. Cover the pork with half of the olive oil. Cook in a hot oven until crunchy and browned, about 20 to 30 minutes.

6. Warm a pan and add the water and stevia to the pan, and add the walnuts once the stevia has dissolved. Cook for five minutes until the liquid has caramelised the walnuts.

7. Tip the nuts onto a tray and leave to cool. Note: they will be hot.

8. Chop the pear and cheese into bite-sized pieces.

9. Make the vinaigrette by adding the mustards, vinegar and oil into a bowl and mixing well.

10. By this time the pork should be cooked. Remove set aside to cool, then chop into bite sized chunks.

11. Toss the salad in the vinaigrette and add the pork, nuts, cheese and pear.

Nutritional Information: Carbs 5g Calories 567 Fat 55g Protein 13g.

34. Cauliflower Taboule Salad

Prep time: 5 minutes

Cooking time

Servings: 1

Ingredients

- 3 oz. Cauliflower florets
- 2 tbsps. Parsley
- 6 mint leaves
- 2 diced tomatoes
- 2 cucumbers
- 6 tbsps. Lemon juice
- 2 tbsps. Olive oil
- Salt
- Pepper

Instructions:

1. Make a couscous-like mass from the cauliflower florets by mincing them.
2. Mix the cauliflower florets with finely cut herbs, tomatoes, lemon, olive oil, salt, and pepper.
3. This tasty fresh salad may be used as a garnish or as the meal itself.

Nutrition Information: Calories per serving: 86 Carbohydrates: 6g, Protein: 2g, Fat: 6g

35. Caprese Salad

You will love this recipe and it will remind you of dish your grandma used to make.

Preparing time:45 minutes

Serves: 5

Ingredients:

Ingredients:

- 3 c. grape tomatoes
- 4 peeled garlic cloves
- 2 tbsp. avocado oil
- 10 pearl-sized mozzarella balls
- 4 c. baby spinach leaves
- ¼ c. fresh basil leaves
- 1 tbsp. of each:
- Brine reserved from the cheese
- Pesto

Directions:

1. Use aluminum foil to cover a baking tray. Program the oven to 400°F. Arrange the cloves and tomatoes on the baking pan and drizzle with the oil.
2. Bake 20-30 minutes until the tops are slightly browned.
3. Drain the liquid (saving one tablespoon) from the mozzarella. Mix the pesto with the brine.
4. Arrange the spinach in a large serving bowl. Transfer the tomatoes to the dish along with the roasted garlic. Drizzle with the pesto sauce.
5. Garnish with the mozzarella balls, and freshly torn basil leaves.

Nutritional Values Per Serving: Calories: 190.75 |63.49 g Fat | Carbohydrates: 4.58 g | Protein: 7.71 g

36. Low-Carb Mayonnaise for the Horseradish Dressing

Preparing time:25 minutes

Serves: 8

Ingredients:

- 1 egg yolk
- 1-2 t. white vinegar/lemon juice
- 1 tbsp. Dijon mustard
- 1 c. light olive oil

Directions

Ahead of time, take out the egg and mustard to become room temperature.

1. Mix the mustard and egg. Slowly, pour the oil until the mixture thickens.
2. Pour in the lemon juice/vinegar. Stir well. Add a pinch of salt and pepper for additional flavoring.

Nutritional Values Per Serving: Calories: 736 | Protein: 41.4 g | Carbohydrates: 6.2 g| Fat: 59.4 g Fiber: 7.3g

37. Vegetarian Club Salad

. Preparing time:25 minutes

Serves: 5

Ingredients:

- 2 tbsp. of each:
- -Mayonnaise
- -Sour cream
- ½ t. of each:
- -Onion powder
- -Garlic powder
- 1 tbsp. milk
- 1 t. dried parsley
- 3 large hard-boiled eggs
- 4 oz. cheddar cheese
- ½ c. cherry tomatoes
- 1 c diced cucumber
- 3 c. torn romaine lettuce
- 1 tbsp. Dijon mustard

Directions:

1. Slice the hard-boiled eggs and cube the cheese. Cut the tomatoes into halves and dice the cucumber.
2. Prepare the dressing (dried herbs, mayo, and sour cream) mixing well.
3. Add one tablespoon of milk to the mixture - and another if it's too thick.

4. Layer the salad with the vegetables, cheese, and egg slices. Scoop a spoonful of mustard in the center along with a drizzle of dressing.

5. Toss and enjoy!

Nutritional Values Per Serving: Calories: 329.67| Fat: 26.32 g| Carbohydrates: 4.83 g| Protein: 16.82 g Fiber: 7.3g

38. Thai Pork Salad

Preparing time:25 minutes

Serves: 5

Ingredients:

- 2 c. romaine lettuce
- 10 oz. pulled pork
- ¼ medium chopped red bell pepper
- ¼ c. chopped cilantro
- Ingredients for the Sauce:
- 2 tbsp. of each:
- -Tomato paste
- -Chopped cilantro
- Juice & zest of 1 lime
- 2 tbsp. (+) 2 t. soy sauce
- 1 t. of each:
- -Red curry paste
- -Five Spice
- -Fish sauce
- ¼ t. red pepper flakes
- 1 tbsp. (+) 1 t. rice wine vinegar
- ½ t. mango extract
- 10 drops liquid stevia

Directions:

1. Zest half of the lime and chop the cilantro.
2. Mix all of the sauce fixings.
3. Blend the barbecue sauce components and set aside.

4. Pull the pork apart and make the salad. Pour a glaze over the pork with a bit of the sauce.

Nutritional Values Per Serving: Calories: 461 | Fat: 32.6 g| Carbohydrates: 5.2 g | Protein: 29.2 g Fiber: 7.3g

39. Egg Salad Stuffed Avocado

Preparing time: 20 minutes

Serves: 5

Ingredients:

- 6 large hard-boiled eggs
- 3 celery ribs
- 1/3 med. red onion
- 4 tbsp. mayonnaise
- 2 tbsp. fresh lime juice
- 2 t. brown mustard
- Pepper & salt to taste
- ½ t. cumin
- 1 t. hot sauce
- 3 med. avocados

Directions:

1. Begin by chopping the onions, celery, and eggs. Discard the pit and slice the avocado in half.
2. Combine with all of the other fixings except for the avocado.
3. Scoop the salad into the avocado and serve!

Nutritional Values Per Serving: Calories: 280.57 | Fat: 24.83 g| Carbohydrates: 3.03 g| Protein: 8.32 g Fiber: 7.3g

40. Bistro Steak Salad with Horseradish Dressing

Preparing time:35 minutes

Serves: 2

Ingredients:

- 1 (12 oz.) rib-eye steak
- ¼ t. of each:
- -Pepper
- -Salt
- 1 (2.1 oz.) small red onion
- 1 (7 oz.) bag romaine salad greens
- 4 slices uncured bacon
- ½ cup (2 oz.) sliced radishes
- oz. cherry tomatoes
- Ingredients for the Dressing:
- 2 tbsp. prepared horseradish
- ¼ c. mayonnaise
- Pepper and salt

Directions

1. Thinly slice the onion and radishes.
2. Place parchment paper on a baking tin. Set the oven temperature to 350°F. Arrange the bacon in a single layer in the pan. Bake for 15 minutes. Drain and break into small pieces.
3. Pat the steak with paper towels. Season with the pepper and salt. Grill for four minutes and flip. Continue cooking another 12-15 minutes (medium is approximately 12 minutes or internal temperature of 155°F.).

4. Let it cool down five minutes, and slice against the grain into small slices.

5. Prepare the dressing and enjoy.

Nutritional Values Per Serving: Calories: 736 | Protein: 41.4 g | Carbohydrates: 6.2 g| Fat: 59.4 g

CHAPTER 19: KETO FISH RECIPES

41. Shrimp Tuscany

Prep time: 0 minutes

Cooking time: 15 minutes

Servings: 4

Ingredients

- Baby kale (.25 c.)
- Sun dried tomatoes (5)
- Parmesan (.5 c.)
- Salt (1 tsp.)
- Dried basil (1 tsp.)
- Crushed garlic cloves (2)
- Whole milk (.5 c.)
- Cream cheese, cubed (1 c.)
- Butter (1 Tbsp.)
- Raw shrimp (1 lb.)

Directions:

1. Melt up the butter in a pan and add in the shrimp. Cook for 30 seconds and then turn them around. Cook until they turn pink.
2. Add in the cream cheese and milk into the pan and increase the heat. Stir so the cheese melts completely.
3. Add in the basil, salt, and garlic and keep cooking. Allow the dish to simmer so that the sauce can thicken.
4. Add in the tomatoes and kale and then serve.

Nutritional Information: Calories: 280 Fats: 18g Carbs: 6.5g Protein: 23g

42. Shrimp in Tuscan Cream Sauce

Prep time: 10 minutes

Cooking time: 5 minutes

Servings: 2

Ingredients

- 1 lb. raw shrimp
- 1 tbsp. butter
- 1 c. cubed cream cheese
- ½ c. whole milk
- 2 cloves garlic
- 1 tsp. dried basil
- 1 tsp. salt
- ½ c. Parmesan
- 5 sun-dried tomatoes
- ¼ c. baby kale

Directions:

1. Melt the butter in a large pan.
2. Add the shrimp and lower the temperature.
3. Cook the shrimp for thirty seconds, then turn them and cook until they are beginning to turn pink.
4. Add the cream cheese.
5. Pour milk into the pan and increase the heat. Stir until the cheese has melted and there are no lumps.
6. Add the garlic, salt and basil and continue stirring.

7. Throw in the cheese, and finish stirring once it has melted in. Leave the dish to simmer until the sauce shows signs of thickening.
8. Finally add the tomatoes and kale.
9. Serve straight away.

Nutritional Information: Calories per serving: 280 Fat: 18, Carbohydrates: 6.5g, Protein: 23g

43.   Almond Pesto Salmon

Preparing time:25 minutes

Serves: 5

Ingredients

- 1 garlic clove
- ¼ c. almonds
- 1 tbsp. olive oil
- ½ lemon
- ½ t. each: Parsley -Pink Himalayan salt
- 2 (6 oz.) Atlantic salmon fillets
- ½ shallot
- 2 handfuls lettuce
- 2 tbsp. butter

Directions

1. Make the Pesto: Pulse the almonds, olive oil, and garlic, in a food processor to form a paste. Combine the parsley, salt, and juice of the lemon. Set to the side.
2. Dry the salmon fillets and season them with a sprinkle of salt and pepper.
3. Cook the salmon four to six minutes (skin side down) in a lightly greased pan. Flip it and butter the pan to baste the fish for a minute or so (rare inside).
4. Serve over some lettuce with a spoonful of pesto, slivered almonds, and shallots.

Nutritional Information: Calories: 610 |Net Carbs: 6 g | Protein: 38 g | Fat: 47 g

44.   Salmon and Potato Salad

Prep time: 10 minutes

Cooking time: 25 minutes

Servings: 6

Ingredients

- Chopped parsley (1 Tbsp.)
- Salmon (6 oz.)
- Chopped onion (1)
- Olive oil (1 Tbsp.)
- Baking potatoes (3)

Instructions:

1. Boil the potatoes and eggs together until done. While those are boiling, heat up some oil in a pan and fry the onions.
2. Place the salmon slices into a dish and put the onions on top.
3. Top with the eggs and he potatoes and sprinkle the parsley on top before serving.

Nutritional Information: Calories: 370 Fat: 30g Carbs: 10g Protein: 15g

45.   Chili Lime Cod

Preparing time:25 minutes

Serves: 5

Ingredients

- 1 (10-12 oz.) wild-caught cod
- 1/3 c. coconut flour
- 1 egg
- 1 lime
- ½ teaspoon cayenne pepper
- 1 t. of each: -Garlic powder -Salt -Crushed red pepper

Directions

1. Program the oven temperature to 400°F.
2. In separate dishes, whip the egg, and remove any lumps from the flour.
3. Let the fillet soak in the egg dish for one minute on each side. Add it to the flour dish, and then add it to a baking sheet.
4. Sprinkle the spices and drizzle the lime juice over the cod.
5. Bake 10 to 12 minutes or when it easily flakes apart.
6. Drizzle with some Sriracha if you wish, and enjoy.

Nutritional information: Calories: 215 |Carbs: 3 g | Protein: 37 g| Fat: 5 g

46.   Mediterranean Tuna

Prep time 15 minutes

Cooking time: 0 minutes

Servings: 6

Ingredients

- Pepper
- Salt
- Red pepper flakes
- Drained capers (1.5 Tbsp.)
- Lemon juice (1.5 Tbsp.)
- Parsley (.33 c.)
- Quartered green olives (.33 c.)
- Roasted red peppers (.75 c.)
- Olive oil (.75 c.)
- Crumbled feta cheese (1.5 c.)
- Tuna (15 oz.)
- Endives (300 grams)

Directions:

1. Add the tuna into a bowl and crumble it around. Fold in the rest of the ingredients, making sure to mix well.
2. Divide this salad into the six servings and then place into airtight containers to eat when ready.

Nutritional Information: Calories: 354 Fats: 26g Carbs: 5g Protein: 25g

47.   Smoked Salmon

Prep time: 10 minutes

Servings: 4

Ingredients

- Salmon caviar (2 Tbsp.)
- Olive oil (1 Tbsp.)
- Pepper
- Creamed horseradish (1 Tbsp.)
- Lemon zest (1)
- Greek yogurt (100g)
- Cream cheese (200g.)
- Smoked salmon (100g)

Instructions:

1. Take out your food blender and add the Greek yogurt, cream cheese, salmon, and lemon zest.

2. Add in the pepper and horseradish as well. Blend these together until nice and smooth.

3. Put this into a bowl and drizzle on the olive oil and salmon caviar and serve.

Nutritional Information: Calories: 298 Fat: 26g Carbs: 2g Protein: 14g

48.   Salmon Fishcakes

It's very delicious, creamy and easy to make! What more could you want?

Prep time: 10 minutes

Cooking time: 5 minutes

Servings: 2

Ingredients

- 2 large eggs
- 4 ounces sliced smoked salmon
- ½ tbsp. butter
- 2 tbsp. fresh chives
- 6 sliced mushrooms
- Salt and Pepper
- Jar of ready-made Hollandaise sauce

Instructions:

1. Boil the eggs for ten to twelve minutes. They need to be hard boiled.
2. Dice the salmon finely while the eggs are cooking.
3. Heat the butter under a high heat. Put half the salmon in to crisp it up, then set aside.
4. Run the eggs under cold water and peel.
5. Mash the eggs using a fork until they are broken up into fine pieces.
6. Take the raw salmon and half of the chives and mix with the egg and two to three tbsp. of Hollandaise sauce.
7. Split the mixture into four lumps and form into rough balls.
8. Mix the crispy salmon and remaining chives together and dip the egg balls into them until fully coated.

Nutritional Information: Calories per serving: 283 Fat: 23g, Carbohydrates: 1g, Protein: 18g

49. Omega-3 Rich Salmon Soup

Total Time: 42 MINS

Serves 8)

Ingredients:

- 2 pounds' salmon fillets
- Two tablespoons coconut oil
- 2 cups carrots, peeled and chopped
- 1 cup celery stalk, cut
- 1 cup yellow onion, chopped
- 2 cups cauliflower, cut
- 4 cups homemade chicken broth
- 1½ cups half-and-half
- ¼ cup fresh parsley, chopped

Directions:

1. Arrange the trivet in the bottom of Instant Pot. Add 1 cup of water in Instant Pot.
2. Place the salmon fillets on top of trivet in a single layer.
3. Secure the lid and cook under "Manual" and "High Pressure" for about 8-9 minutes.
4. Select the "Cancel" and carefully do a Quick release.
5. Remove the lid and transfer the salmon onto a plate.
6. Cut the salmon into bite-sized pieces.
7. Remove water and trivet from Instant Pot.
8. Select the "Cancel" and stir in the cauliflower and broth.
9. Secure the lid and cook under "Manual" and "High Pressure" for about 8 minutes.
10. Select the "Cancel" and carefully do a Natural release.

11. Remove the lid and stir in salmon pieces, half-and-half, salt and black pepper until well combined.

12. Serve immediately with the garnishing of parsley.

Nutritional Information per Serving: Calories: 284 Fat: 16.4g Saturated Fat: 7.4g Sodium: 508mg Carbohydrates: 8.3g Dietary Fiber: 1.9g Sugar: 3.2g Protein: 26.8g

50. Special Occasion's Crab Legs

(Total Time: 25 MIN| Serves: 8)

Ingredients:

- 1½ pounds frozen crab legs
- Salt, to taste
- Two tablespoons butter, melted

Directions:

1. Arrange the trivet in the bottom of Instant Pot. Add 1 cup of water and about teaspoon of salt in Instant Pot.
2. Place the crab legs on top of trivet and sprinkle with salt.
3. Secure the lid and cook under "Manual" and "High Pressure" for about 4 minutes.
4. Select the "Cancel" and carefully do a Quick release.
5. Remove the lid and transfer crab legs onto a serving platter.
6. Drizzle with butter and serve.

Nutritional Information per Serving: Calories: 297 Fat: 11.1g Saturated Fat: 4.9g Carbohydrates: 0g Dietary Fiber: 0g Sugar: 0g Protein: 43.6g

CHAPTER 20: KETO MEATS RECIPES

51. Beefy Pizza

Preparing time:35 minutes

Serves: 4

Ingredients:

- 2 large eggs
- 1 pkg. (20 oz.) ground beef
- 28 pepperoni slices
- ½ c. of each:
- Shredded cheddar cheese
- Pizza sauce
- 4 oz. mozzarella cheese
- Also Needed: 1 Cast iron skillet

Directions

1. Combine the eggs, beef, and seasonings and place in the skillet to form the crust.
2. Bake until the meat is done or about 15 minutes.
3. Take it out and add the sauce, cheese, and toppings. Remove and enjoy!

Nutritional information per serving Calories: 610| Net Carbs: 2 g | Protein: 44 g | Fat: 45 g Fiber: 7.3g

52. Bacon Cheeseburger Casserole

Preparing time:25 minutes

Servings: 6

Ingredients

- bacon slices
- 1 lb. lean ground beef
- ½ c. almond flour
- 2 ½ c. riced cauliflower
- ½ t. of each: Onion powder -Garlic powder
- 1 tbsp. Psyllium husk powder
- 2 tbsp. of each: Ketchup – reduced-sugar -Mayonnaise
- 1 tbsp. Dijon mustard
- large eggs
- Pepper and salt to taste
- oz. cheddar cheese – divided

Directions

1. Prepare the oven setting to 350°F.
2. In a food processor; rice the cauliflower and add the dry ingredients.
3. Toss in the bacon and ground beef. Pulse until it's a bit pasty and crumbly. Cook the mixture over the med-high setting on the stove.
4. Combine all of the components in a mixing dish and add ½ of the cheese.

   Press into the parchment paper-lined pan and top it off with the rest of the cheese.
5. Bake 25-30 minutes on the top oven rack. Let it cool about five to ten minutes before serving.

Nutritional Information per Serving: Calories: 478 | Protein: 32.2 g | Net Carbs: 3.6 g | Fat: 35.5 g

53.   Pan-Fried Chops

Preparing time:25 minutes

Serves: 5

Ingredients

- ½ c. coconut flour
- 1 t. of each:
- ¼ t. cayenne pepper
- 1 tbsp. butter
- pork chops – bone-in

Directions

1. Mix all the dry components in a bowl. Rinse and pat dry the chops and coat with the mixture.
2. Warm up the butter in a skillet. Add the chops and fry for four to five minutes on each side.
3. Serve with a salad (add the carbs).

Nutritional Information per Serving: Calories: 298 | Protein: 27 g | Carbs: 4 g | Fat: 15 g

54. Balsamic Beef Roast

Preparing time:25 minutes

Serves: 5

Ingredients

- 1 boneless (approx. 3 lb.) chuck roast
- 1 t. of each: Garlic powder -Black ground pepper
- 1 tbsp. kosher salt
- ¼ c. balsamic vinegar
- ½ c. chopped onion
- 2 c. water
- ¼ t. xanthan gum
- Garnish Ingredients: Freshly chopped parsley

Directions

1. Combine the garlic powder, salt, and pepper. Use the mixture to rub the chuck roast.
2. Prepare a heavy skillet and sear the roast. Add the vinegar and deglaze the pan as you continue cooking for one more minute.
3. Toss the onion into a pot with the (two cups) boiling water along with the roast. Cover with a top and simmer for three to four hours on a low setting.
4. Take the meat from the pot and add to a cutting surface. Shred into chunks and remove any fat or bones.
5. Add the xanthan gum to the broth and whisk. Place the roasted meat back in the pan to warm up.
6. Serve with a favorite side dish.

Nutritional Information per Serving: Calories: 393| Protein: 30 g | Net Carbs: 3 g | Fat: 28 g

55.   Bacon & BBQ Cheeseburger Waffles

Preparing time: 10 minutes

Servings: 4

Ingredients for the Waffles

- 1 ½ oz. cheddar cheese
- 1 c. cauliflower crumbles
- 2 large eggs
- ¼ t. of each: -Onion powder -Garlic powder
- tbsp. grated parmesan cheese
- tbsp. almond flour
- Pepper and salt to your liking
- Ingredients for the Toppings
- oz. lean ground beef
- tbsp. barbecue sauce – sugar-free
- 4 bacon slices
- 1 ½ oz. cheddar cheese
- To Taste: Salt and pepper

Directions

1. Shred all of the cheese and divide into two bowls.
2. Combine the eggs, ½ of the cheddar cheese, spices, flour, and parmesan cheese.
3. Prepare the bacon on the stove using the med-high setting. When done toss in the beef and cook until done (set aside for step 5). Add the excess of grease into the waffle mixture (step 2). Make a thick paste with the blender.
4. Add ½ of the mix into the waffle iron and repeat with the remainder of the mix.

5. Add the barbecue sauce to the ground beef and bacon mixture in the pan.

6. For each waffle, add ½ of the beef, and ½ of the cheese on top. Broil for one to two minutes until the cheese melts.

7. Serve and enjoy immediately.

Calories: 405.25 | Protein: 18.8 g | Net Carbs: 4.35 g | Fat: 33.94 g

56.   **Cumin Spiced Beef Wraps**

Preparing time: 10 minutes

Servings: 2

Ingredients

- 1-2 tbsp. coconut oil
- ¼ onion – diced
- 2/3 lb. ground beef
- 2 tbsp. chopped cilantro
- 1 diced red bell pepper
- 1 t. minced ginger/2 t. cumin
- minced garlic cloves
- Pepper and salt to your liking
- 8 large cabbage leaves

Directions

1. Heat up a frying pan and pour in the oil. Saute the peppers, onions, and ground beef using medium heat. When done, add the pepper, salt, cumin, ginger, cilantro, and garlic.
2. Add the water (¾ full) to a stockpot and wait for it to boil. Cook each leaf for 20 seconds, plunge it in cold water and drain before placing it on your serving dish.
3. Scoop the mixture onto each leaf, fold, and enjoy.

Nutritional Information per Serving: Calories: 375 |Net Carbs: 4 g | Protein: 30 g | Fat: 26 g

57.   Ground Beef Stir Fry

Preparing time: 10 minutes

Servings: 3

Ingredients

- 10 ½ oz. ground beef
- med. brown mushrooms
- ½ c. broccoli
- 2 leaves kale
- ½ med. Spanish onion
- 1 tbsp. coconut oil
- ½ med. red pepper
- 1 tbsp. of each: -Cayenne pepper -Chinese Five Spices

Directions

1. Prepare the veggies. Chop the broccoli and slice the mushrooms.
2. Warm up a skillet using the med-high heat setting. Pour in the oil and onions and cook for a minute.
3. Combine the remainder of the vegetables and cook an additional two minutes—stir frequently.
4. Mix in the spices and beef. Reduce the temperature setting to medium and continue cooking for approximately two more minutes.
5. Stir and put a top on the skillet and continue cooking for five or ten more minutes.

Nutritional Information per Serving: Calories: 307 | Protein: 29 g | Carbs: 7 g | Fat: 18.0 g

58. Chicken Fried Pork Chops

Preparing time: 45 minutes

Serves: 4

Ingredients:

- 1 oz. ground pork rinds
- 1 tbsp. chopped nuts
- 2 tbsp. of each:
- -Flaxseed meal
- -Almond flour
- 1 t. salt
- 1 large egg
- 4 tbsp. fat/oil – your choice
- 4 medium (bone-out 16 oz. ea.) pork chops

Directions

1. Combine the flaxseed meal, flour, and nut blend.
2. Warm up the oil/fat in a skillet using the med-hi setting.
3. Whisk an egg in a dish and dip the chop. Dip in the rind mixture (step 1). Coat well and fry for about four to five minutes for each side. The internal temperature should reach 145°F.
4. Serve and enjoy!

Nutritional information per serving Calories: 390 | Protein: 28.8 g | Carbs: 0.8 g | Fat: 20.8 g Fiber: 7.3g

59. Parmesan Crusted Pork Chops

Preparing time:15 minutes

Serves: 4)

Ingredients:

- 6 oz. parmesan cheese
- 14 pork chops
- 2 large eggs
- ¾ c. almond flour
- Pepper and salt – if desired
- For Frying: Bacon grease

Directions

1. Warm up the oven to 400°F.
2. Grate the parmesan and mix with the flour and spices.
3. Whisk the eggs in a shallow dish.
4. Dip the chops in the eggs; then the parmesan mixture.
5. Fry in the bacon grease on each side for one minute.
6. Arrange on a baking dish in the oven, baking until done.

Nutritional information per serving Calories: 354|Net Carbs: 3 g | Protein: 33 g | Fat: 34 g Fiber: 7.3g

60. Beef Burritos

Preparing time:35 minutes

Serves: 8

Ingredients:

For the Beef:

- 2 lbs. of sirloin steak
- 1 cup of chicken soup or broth (canned works well)
- 1 cup of BBQ sauce
- ½ of an onion, chopped up roughly
- 2 tsp of salt
- ½ tsp of black pepper
- 5 fresh cloves of garlic, crushed
- 1/2 tsp of cinnamon
- 2 bay leaves

For the Taco

- 8 low carb wraps
- ½ cup of mayo
- 1 ½ cups of coleslaw (you can make your own, but ready brought works just as well)

Directions:

1. Pat dry the sirloin with paper towels, and score along the sides.
2. Combine the salt, pepper and cinnamon. Sprinkle it evenly onto the steak, making sure that there is an even covering.

3. Put the onion and garlic in the slow cooker. Place the beef on top and cover with the soup. Add the bay leaves and cook for eight hours.
4. When cooked, remove and strain the ingredients. Then shred the beef mix by pulling it with two forks.
5. Add the BBQ sauce and combine everything well.
6. Put some of the beef into the wrap, add coleslaw and dash of mayo. Wrap and eat.

Nutritional Information(per serving) Carbs 14g Calories 750 Fat 50g Protein 60g Fiber: 7.3g

CHAPTER 21: KETO DESSERTS

61. Mini Chocolate Cakes

Preparing time: 35 minutes

Serves: 2

Ingredients:

- 2 tbsp heavy cream
- ¼ c baking cocoa
- ½ tsp baking powder
- 2 tbsp Splenda
- One tsp vanilla
- Two eggs

Directions:

1. Stir everything together in a bowl. Grease two ramekins and split the batter between the two.
2. Place a cup of water to the pot and set in the trivet.
3. Set the ramekins and lock the lid in place the set the cooker on high for nine minutes.
4. Quick release the pressure and then flip the cakes onto a plate.

Nutrition Information per Serving: Calories: 120 Protein: .8g Carbohydrates: 7g net Fat: 4.8g Fiber: 7.3g

63. Ricotta Lemon Cheesecake

Preparing time:25 minutes

Serves: 6

Ingredients:

- Two eggs
- ½ tsp lemon extract
- One lemon, juice and zest
- 1/3 c ricotta
- ¼ c trivia
- 8 oz cream cheese
- Topping:
- One tsp Truvia
- 2 tbsp sour cream

Directions:

1. Beat all the ingredients together except for the eggs until there are no lumps. Mix the eggs. Don't overbeat. Pour this into a greased springform pan and place foil over the top.
   2. Add two cups of water and the trivet in your pot and set on the cake. Lock the lid and set to high for 30 minutes. Let pressure release naturally.
   3. Stir together the Truvia and sour cream. Spread this over the warm cake and refrigerate for six to eight hours.

Nutrition Information per Serving: Calories: 190 Protein: 8g Carbohydrates: 6g net Fat: 9g Fiber: 7.3g

64. Wheat Belly Yogurt

Preparing time:20 minutes

Serves: 4

Ingredients:

- 2 tbsp. full-fat yogurt with live cultures
- 16 oz. heavy whipping cream

Directions:

1. Stir the ingredients together in a glass bowl.
2. Place in your Instant Pot and follow the yogurt making Directions.

Nutrition Information per Serving: Calories: 149 Protein: 8.5g Carbohydrates: 7g net Fat: 8g Fiber: 7.3g

65. Eggs in a Cup

Preparing time: 5 minutes

Serves: 4

Ingredients:

- Pepper and salt
- ¼ c half & half
- 2 tbsp. cilantro
- ½ c cheddar cheese
- ½ c shredded cheese
- 1 c diced veggies
- Four eggs

Directions:

1. Combine the coriander, pepper, salt, half & half, cheese, vegetables, and eggs and divide into four-pint jars. Loosely place on lids.
2. Add two cups water to the pot and trivet. Set the jars. Lock the lid and set the cooker on high for five minutes. Once done, release the pressure.
3. Add other cheese and broil for a few minutes.

Nutrition Information per Serving: Calories: 115 Protein: 9g Carbohydrates: 2g net Fat: 9g Fiber: 7.3g

66. Vanilla Bean Cheesecake

Preparing time:10 minutes

Serves: 8

Ingredients:

- Raspberry jam
- One vanilla bean, scraped
- ½ c swerve
- One tsp vanilla
- Two eggs
- 16 oz cultured cream cheese

Directions:

1. Whisk everything together in a blender. Add to a spring form pan and cover with foil. Add two cups of water to the pot and set on a rack.
2. Ease in the pan and lock the lid then set the cooker on high for 20 minutes. Once done, naturally release pressure.
3. Take out of the pot and let it cool to room temp. Refrigerate at least an hour before serving.

Nutrition Information per Serving: Calories: 100 Protein: 6g Carbohydrates: 8g net Fat: 10g Fiber: 7.3g

70. Pumpkin Pecan Cake

Preparing time: 20 minutes

Serves: **10**

Ingredients:

- ¼ tsp salt
- One tsp ginger
- ¼ c protein powder
- Four eggs
- 1 c pumpkin puree
- ¼ tsp cloves
- One tsp vanilla
- 1 ½ tsp cinnamon
- ¼ c butter, melted
- Two tsp baking powder
- 1/3 c coconut flour
- ¾ c swerve
- 1 ½ c raw pecan

Directions:

1. Grease your pot, then grind pecans in a processor. Place in a bowl and mix the spices, sweetener, and coconut.
2. Mix the vanilla, butter, eggs, and pumpkin.
3. Spread into the pot. Place the lid and set to slow cook for 2 ½ hours. Enjoy.

Nutrition Information per Serving: Calories: 250 Protein: 7g Carbohydrates: 8g net Fat: 17g Fiber: 7.3g

71. Chocolate Cream

Preparing time: 10 minutes

Serves: 4

Ingredients:

- Two heavy cream
- ¼ cup unsweetened dark chocolate, chopped
- Three eggs
- One tsp orange zest
- One tsp stevia powder
- One tsp vanilla extract
- ½ tsp salt

Directions:

1. Plug in your instant pot and press the 'Saute' button. Add heavy cream, chopped chocolate, stevia powder, vanilla extract, orange zest, and salt. Stir well and simmer until the chocolate has completely melted.
2. Press the 'Cancel' button and crack eggs, one at the time, stirring constantly. Remove from the instant pot.
3. Transfer the mixture to 4 mason jars with loose lids.
4. Pour 2 cups of water in your instant pot and set the trivet in the stainless steel insert. Add jars and seal the lid.
5. Set the steam release handle and press the 'Manual' button. Set the timer for 10 minutes.
6. When done, perform a quick release by moving the steam valve to the 'Venting' position.
7. Open the lid and remove the jars. Chill to room temperature and then transfer to the refrigerator.

8. Top with some whipped cream before serving.

Nutritional information per Serving (Calories 267 | Total Fats 26.2g | Net Carbs: 2.4g | Protein 5.6g |Fiber: 0.2g)

72. Butter Pancakes

Preparing time: 10 minutes

Serves: 6)

Ingredients:

- 2 cups cream cheese
- 2 cups almond flour
- Six large eggs
- ¼ tsp salt
- 2 tbsp. butter
- ¼ tsp ground ginger
- ½ tsp cinnamon powder

Directions

1. Mix cream cheese, butter and eggs
2. Slowly add flour beating continually.
3. Finally, add salt, ginger, and cinnamon. Continue to beat until fully incorporated.
4. Plug in your instant pot and press the 'Saute' button. Grease the stainless steel insert with the remaining butter and heat up.
5. Pour in about ½ cup of the batter and cook for 2-3 minutes or until golden color. Repeat the process with the remaining dough.
6. Serve warm.

Per Serving (Calories 432 | Total Fats 40.2g | Net Carbs: 3.5g | Protein 14.2g |Fiber: 1g)

73. Raspberry Cookies

Preparing time: 15 minutes

Serves: 6

Ingredients:

- 1 ½ cup almond flour
- ¾ tsp baking powder
- ¼ tsp baking soda
- ¼ cup unsweetened almond milk
- 2 large eggs
- ¼ cup almond butter
- ¼ cup Swerve
- 1 tbsp. raw almonds, chopped
- One tsp raspberry extract

Directions:

1. Beat eggs and raspberry extract and swerve gently pour in the milk and almond butter. Continue to beat for 1 minute.
2. Finally, add the remaining ingredients and mix until thoroughly combined.
3. Line some parchment paper over a small baking dish and plug in your instant pot. Pour in 1 cup of water and set the trivet at the bottom of the steel insert.
4. Spoon one tablespoon of the mixture onto the prepared baking pan and flatten the surface with your hands.
5. Loosely cover with some aluminum foil and seal the lid. Set the steam release handle to the 'Sealing' position and press the 'Manual' button. Set the timer for 15 minutes.

6. When you hear the cooker's end signal, perform a quick release and open the lid.

7. Remove the pan and transfer cookies to a wire rack to cool completely before serving.

Nutritional information Per Serving (Calories 78 | Total Fats 6g | Net Carbs: 1.4g | Protein 4g |Fiber: 1g)

74. Vanilla Mousse with Chocolate Sauce

Preparing time: 20 minutes

Serves: 4

Ingredients:

- 2 cups cream cheese
- 1 cup whipped cream
- 4 tbsp. coconut oil
- One tsp vanilla extract
- ¼ cup Swerve
- 4 tbsp. unsweetened cocoa powder
- ¼ cup unsweetened dark chocolate
- ¼ cup unsweetened almond milk

Directions:

1. In a container, combine cream cheese, whipped cream, two tablespoons of coconut oil, cocoa powder, vanilla extract, and swerve. With a paddle attachment on, beat well on high speed until light and fluffy mixture. Divide between 4 serving cups and refrigerate.
2. Grease the stainless steel insert with the remaining coconut oil and heat up. Add chocolate and gently melt, stirring constantly. Pour in the milk and simmer for 5 minutes.
3. Press the cancel button and remove the chocolate sauce. Drizzle the chilled mousse with the sauce and serve immediately.

Nutritional information Per Serving (Calories 653 | Total Fats 66.3g | Net Carbs: 5.2g | Protein 10.2g |Fiber: 0.8g)

75. Sweet Almond Buns

Preparing time:20 minutes

Serves: 6

Ingredients:

- 1 cup almond flour
- ½ cup coconut flour
- 1/3 cup psyllium husk powder
- ½ cup cocoa powder, unsweetened
- One tsp baking soda
- Four large eggs
- 1 tbsp. raw almonds, finely chopped
- ½ cup Swerve
- ½ cup almond butter

Directions:

1. Mix all the dry ingredients and add eggs, one at the time, and beat well with a dough hook attachment. Now add almond butter and continue to beat until smooth dough.

2. Transfer the dough to a lightly floured surface and divide into six equal balls. Press each ball with your hands until about 1-inch thick. Set aside.

3. Line some parchment paper over a small baking pan and plug in your instant pot. Pour in 1 cup of water and place the trivet at the bottom.

4. Gently place the buns in your baking pan and loosely cover with aluminum foil. Place the pan in the pot and seal the lid. Set the steam release handle to the 'Sealing' position and press the 'Manual' button.

5. Set the timer for 30 minutes.

6. When done, release the pressure naturally for 15 minutes and then move the pressure valve to the 'Venting' position to release any remaining tension.

7. Open the lid and remove the pan. Cool to room temperature and transfer buns to a wire rack to cool completely.

Nutritional information Per Serving (Calories 130 | Total Fats 8.2g | Net Carbs: 4.2g | Protein 7.7g |Fiber: 6.1g)

76. Cocoa Patties

Preparing time:25 minutes

Serves: 4

Ingredients:

- 1 cup cream cheese
- Four large eggs
- 2 tbsp. swerve
- ¼ cup cocoa powder, unsweetened
- 2 tbsp. coconut oil plus more for frying
- One tsp vanilla extract

Directions:

1. Mix all the ingredients. With a paddle attachment on, beat well on high speed until thoroughly combined.
2. Plug in your instant pot and press the 'Saute' button. Grease the stainless steel insert with some oil and heat up.
3. Pour in about ¼ cup of the cocoa butter and cook for 3-4 minutes, or until golden-brown color.
4. Optionally, top with some whipped cream.

Nutritional information Per Serving (Calories 456 | Total Fats 45.6g | Net Carbs: 2.1g | Protein 10.7g |Fiber: 0g)

77. Easy Almond Bars

Preparing time: 20 minutes

Serves:

Ingredients:

- One ¼ cup almond flour
- ¼ cup coconut flour
- ½ cup coconut oil
- 2 tbsp. almond butter
- ¼ tsp salt
- 3 tbsp. swerve
- One tsp vanilla extract
- Two large eggs

Directions:

1. Plug in your instant pot and set the trivet. Pour in 1 cup of water at the bottom of the stainless steel insert and set aside.
2. Combine the ingredients in a food processor and process until 'sandy' texture.
3. Line a small baking pan with some parchment paper and add the dough. Press well with the palm of your hands and gently place in your instant pot.
4. Cover with some parchment paper and seal the lid. Set the steam release handle to the 'Sealing' position and press the 'Manual' button.
5. Set the timer for 15 minutes.
6. When done, release the pressure naturally and open the lid. Using oven mitts carefully remove the pan from your instant pot and chill to room temperature.

7. Slice into 6 bars and refrigerate for at least an hour before serving.

Nutritional information Per Serving (Calories 253 | Total Fats 25.7g | Net Carbs: 1.5g | Protein 4.6g |Fiber: 1.4g)

78. Pumpkin Pie Pancakes

Preparing time:25 minutes

Serves: 4

Ingredients:

- 1 cup pumpkin puree
- Three large eggs
- 2 tbsp. swerve
- ¾ cup almond flour
- 4 tbsp. almond milk, unsweetened
- One tsp pumpkin pie seasoning
- ¼ tsp salt
- Two tsp baking powder

Directions:

1. In a large mixing bowl, combine eggs, swerve, pumpkin pie seasoning, and almond milk.
2. With a whisking attachment on, beat well on high speed. Gradually add flour, salt, baking powder, and pumpkin pie seasoning.
3. Continue to mix for another 2 minutes.
4. Finally, add the pumpkin puree and mix well again.
5. Plug in your instant pot and press the 'Saute' button. Grease the stainless steel insert with some oil and heat up. Add about ¼ cup of the batter and cook for 3 minutes.

Nutritional information Per Serving (Calories 143 | Total Fats 10g | Net Carbs: 5.7g | Protein 6.9g |Fiber: 2.7

79. Coconut Brownies with Raspberries

Preparing time:30 minutes

Serves: 6

Ingredients:

- 1 ½ cup almond flour
- ½ cup fresh raspberries
- ½ cup shredded coconut
- ¼ cup Swerve
- One tsp baking soda
- ½ cup coconut oil
- Two large eggs

Directions:

1. Combine almond flour, shredded coconut, baking soda, and swerve. Mix well and add coconut oil and eggs. With a dough hook attachment, beat well until thoroughly combined. Fold in raspberries and set aside.
2. Line a small baking pan with some parchment paper and add the mixture. Press well with your hands and tightly wrap with aluminum foil.
3. Plug in your instant pot and pour in 1 cup of water. Set the trivet and place the baking pan on top.
4. Seal the lid and set the steam release handle. Press the 'Manual' button and set the timer for 20 minutes.
5. When you hear the cooker's end signal, perform a quick release and open the lid.
6. Remove the baking pan and cool completely before slicing.
7. Optionally, sprinkle with some more shredded coconut.

Nutritional information Per Serving (Calories 251 | Total Fats 25.5g | Net Carbs: 1.9g | Protein 4g |Fiber: 2g)

80. Chocolate Chip Cookies

Preparing time:30 minutes

Serves: 10

Ingredients:

- ½ cup almond flour
- ¼ cup flax meal
- ¼ cup coconut flour
- ½ cup almond butter
- ¼ cup coconut oil
- ¼ tsp salt
- ¼ cup Swerve
- Three large eggs
- One tsp vanilla extract
- ¼ cup dark chocolate chips, unsweetened

Directions:

1. Mix all the dry ingredients and Transfer to a food processor along with almond butter, coconut oil, eggs, and vanilla extract. Process until sandy texture.
2. Transfer the mixture to a lightly floured work surface and fold in chocolate chips. Knead with your hands and shape ten balls.
3. Line a baking pan with some parchment paper and place cookies. Plug in your instant pot and pour in 1 cup of water. Set the trivet and place the pan on top.
4. Seal the lid and set the steam release handle to the 'Sealing' position. Press the 'Manual' button and set the timer for 15 minutes.
5. When done, release the pressure naturally and open the lid.

6. Transfer cookies to a wire rack and cool completely before serving.

Nutritional information Per Serving (Calories 133 | Total Fats 11.2g | Net Carbs: 3.2g | Protein 4.2g |Fiber: 3g)

CONCLUSION

Thank you again for purchasing this book!

I hope this book was able to help you to understand how to lose weight while on a ketogenic diet. The next step is to implement what you have learned.

Thank you and good luck in your Ketogenic diet journey.

Lightning Source UK Ltd.
Milton Keynes UK
UKHW021842250621
386185UK00002B/210